I had been on four different pills to control high blood pressure and high cholesterol, plus a drug for constant acid reflux. While following Jason's advice I lost 29 kg, went off all medication, I don't snore any more and my asthma is gone! I honestly believe Jason saved my life.

Lincoln Cobham, CEO, on thelifeplan®, Auckland, October 2011

This is a really useful book; I wish all my patients could read it. I thoroughly enjoyed it and found it hard to put down. I love your summaries and your golden rules. Your book is inspiring and empowering.

Dr Mimi Thomas, GP, Auckland, 2010

I followed your great advice about feeling sluggish and other suggestions, and have felt great since, and also dropped 25 kg! A huge change of life! Keep up the great work.

Maxine, retailer, Waikato, 2011

Without going into all my medical details, I am feeling far more healthy, energetic, fit and happy at 47 than I did at 21, and I don't need my asthma medication. I don't crave junk food. I love the taste of healthy food now. Once you have been exposed to what Jason has discovered, you will be empowered to be aware of how what you eat affects how you feel, and make adjustments and choices to enable you to get the most out of your life.

As a life insurance adviser I am privy to a lot of people's medical history and get to deliver medical report cards to a lot of people. I see a lot of medical and life-quality issues that could be improved through people having better information on which to base their diet and lifestyle decisions. This is what Jason's work provides.

Before reading this book there should be a warning saying, 'Beware contains information that can leave you with EXPLOSIVE energy!'

David, September 2013

Jason just gets better with age. I am sure he looks younger AND more vibrant every time I see him. Upon looking at a photo of Jason and his 21-year-old-son Trey, I embarrassingly could not tell who was father and who was son!

Marg Hardy, Hardys Healthy Living Stores, Hamilton, 2011

I think it's a splendid book! A wonderful piece of work.

My darling Granny Amy, 103 years old, England,
March 2010 (she was not biased at all ...)

I hit 45 and was the wrong side of 125 kg. On top of that I have an eight-year-old daughter who was eating the same bad food as me, and I was aware she was going to start having health problems if I didn't get my act together. On top of that I wasn't fit enough to be the dad I wanted to be with her. Halfway through the year I was diagnosed with type II diabetes, with blood measurements at 52. Something had to change. After one simple six-day vegetable juice fast, I'd shed 6.5 kg, no longer had diabetes, had more energy than I knew what to do with, started sleeping better and felt my mind was sharper than it'd been for a long time at work. The next visit to my doctor had her completely perplexed. Expecting to having to start dispensing drugs to control blood pressure, cholesterol and diabetes in the next few years, all she could ask was 'Stu, you have gone from 52 down to 47, what have you changed? I don't understand these latest results.' Life changing – there's no other way to describe Jason's work. I look forward to seeing how I am in six months.

Stu Colson, Auckland, December 2013

A really good read, great research, inspiring, hard to put down ... a bestseller in the making!

Philip Dowling, Head of Naturopathy, Wellpark College of
Natural Therapies, Auckland, 2012

I will be recommending this book to all my patients.

Dr Eva Tombs, MD, Scotland, 2012

I was diagnosed with atherosclerosis in November 2011 and wrote to you for your advice. I stuck to a plant-based wholefood diet, and made the conscious decision not to take statins. Recently I had all my heart tests again, including an ultrasound where I could see my heart on the screen; we had monitored progress over a two year period. Imagine the thrill of finding that the plaque in my arteries has lessened considerably, the threat of heart disease has been minimised and being told that by continuing my current health ideals there is no above average risk of heart disease in my future. I was so happy I cried. I will never be able to thank you and Tracey enough for your guidance, support and advice.

Cheree on thelifeplan®, November 2013

After working with Jason I have gone from almost 100 kg to under 80 kg. I am heading towards a normal BMI for the first time since my early 20s. My chronic hayfever is gone and I have taken no antihistamines for over 12 months. I have cured my chronic constipation, my haemorrhoids have disappeared and my blood pressure is back to normal.

Maurice on thelifeplan®, September 2013

I have lost 14 kg since starting work with Jason in May 2013. I have been able to discontinue my blood pressure medication and Losec, and I have stopped all daily antihistamines. My cholesterol dropped from a 6 to 5 in one month. My family and friends have asked how I have lost the weight and improved my health so dramatically. Thanks again, you are making a difference to the lives of many people.

Brian on thelifeplan®, November 2013

Eat Less, Live Long

GET HEALTHY, LOSE WEIGHT AND PREVENT DISEASE WITH REGULAR INTELLIGENT FASTING®

Jason Shon Bennett

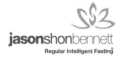

jasonshonbennett
Regular Intelligent Fasting

Published by Jason Shon Bennett, www.jasonshonbennett.com

ISBN 978-0-473-26795-7
Ebook ISBN 978-0-473-26796-4

Publishing services by Oratia Media, www.oratiamedia.com
Images pages 213 and 214, www.shutterstock.com

First published 2014
Second reprint 2014

Printed by Ligare Australia

I dedicate this book to my incredible family. I am, truly, the luckiest man on Planet Earth. My family have missed having as much of me as they would have liked over the last eight years, as I grabbed moments to write. They gave me the time and space to research, study and write when I could have been with them. This book goes out to my four beautiful children, Trey, Tove, Luke and Joel, who inspire me to be a better person every day, and to the absolute love of my life, my soulmate, Tracey.

Without you I could not have done this; I would have folded long ago, I would have crashed and burned, I would have failed; but you held me up when I fell, you caught me when I stumbled, and you supported me when my head was low.

Thank you for your unconditional love and support.

Jason

Disclaimer

I personally think this information will change your life for the better. However, the information presented here is general health advice within the public domain and is meant for people looking for dietary information and basic health improvements.

This information collates and collects hundreds of scientific studies on health, most of which are widely available through the mainstream press/media or the Internet. I am not a medical practitioner, nor is this information, in any way, promising to prevent, mitigate, diagnose or cure any disease condition. Nothing here should be viewed as a substitute for competent healthcare advice from a professional; in fact, I recommend you always seek good and competent advice from a trusted and experienced health professional.

This information should be used in conjunction with the guidance and care of your healthcare practitioner, who should be aware of all medical conditions that you may have, your family history, as well as the medications or supplements you may be taking. This information is for reference and informational purposes only and is not intended as medical counselling or medical advice.

I hereby disclaim any and all responsibility for any loss, injury, damage or expense directly or indirectly arising out of or relating to use or reliance on this information or the material contained here. The reader assumes all risks from the use, non-use or misuse of any information in this book. Most of the information here applies to the healthy population in general; however, not everyone has the same body type, nor does everybody react the same way to the same foods. This information contains sensible and logical dietary advice to help you remain healthy. Everyone is unique and, therefore, everyone has a slightly different nutritional requirement.

As the great Viktoras Kulvinskas said, 'This book itself is of low nutritional content and should never be eaten, only digested.'

Contents

1

I know what it is like to be sick, really sick

In my youth, I was very sick. I was told countless times how my illness was 'incurable' and how I had 'bad genes.' Now, I am very well. Don't buy into the cynical diagnosis that your only option is disease and drugs. Most modern diseases have nothing to do with genetics. You can change how your genes express themselves. You can change your health; you can feel better, lighter, healthier and more alive. You could add 40 happy years to your lifespan. You can live longer. You can transform your life and feel reborn. You can keep up with your children and grandchildren and play, play, play ... The only questions are: do you want it bad enough, and are you willing to do what it takes?'

Jason Shon Bennett (JSB)

Sick, sick, sick

I know what it is like to be sick, really sick. The kind of sick where you think you are going to die and just getting through the hour, or the day, is all you can focus on. When you get that sick it takes over your life. It means that everything you do goes through the 'can I do it?' or 'will I be okay?' filter, until you get to the point where you question your ability in almost all areas of your life. Your experience of being alive is dominated and limited by your sickness.

When you are sick to the point of it being a disability, you are busy trying to stop dying, rather than busy being alive. Your ability and potential is dulled, and the cost of the illness dominates your creativity, energy, expectations, experiences and choices. Everyone has some health issues, be they minor or all-encompassing, but when you are as healthy as you can be, then you have the ability to do anything.

Someone once said that people want more money, time or prestige. What this book offers is more health. Being genuinely healthy is the single most important thing in life, as it gives you the freedom to be anything you want to be, to do anything to which you set your mind and to travel anywhere you like. To come from my level of sickness and medication to the health I have now shows what can be achieved through commitment to and consistency of simple dietary changes. It also shows the incredible healing power of the human body. My experience with extreme poor health and my return to extreme good health has given me my focus in life, my passion and my calling (apart from my love of family, friends, fun, music, movies and mayhem!).

> What we have is a science of illness.
> What we need is a science of health.
>
> Rene Dubos

My Mission   To educate, motivate and inspire change that will transform the health, vitality and longevity of people all over the world.

My Vision   A healthy world, where living to 100+ years old in great health and vitality, without drugs or medical intervention, is seen as normal and expected.

My Expertise   Longevity, fasting, wholefoods and nutrition. The transformation of your digestive, bowel and immune system, the return to high energy levels, the rebuilding of your body to optimum health, and the conscious prevention of modern lifestyle diseases.

> We blindly accepted that the Western way of life was better.
>
> Dr Xu Guangwei, head of the Beijing-based
> China Anti-Cancer Association

The process I propose is one way to get your health back. I do not profess for a moment that my way is the right way, or the only way. It is simply a choice. It has completely transformed my health, cured me and made a dramatic, positive difference for thousands of people I have worked with over nearly 30 years.

The smallest changes to your daily routine can result in the most profound and powerful improvements to your health. This is where I can help. My aim is to educate, elucidate and inspire you to see foods for what they are: the immediate and most powerful solution to all your health issues. Foods are the single most influential factor in your energy levels, your skin, your vitality, your aging and your longevity. Charles Remington said, 'Food is not the problem, food is the solution.'

So, how did I get started down this road? Well, let's go way back to the year that The Beatles (The World's Best Ever Band™) launched an insignificant album called *Sgt. Peppers Lonely Hearts Club Band* ...

My story

Everyone is weird once you get to know them, and I am certainly no exception. I was born by Caesarean section, two months premature, as my mother had developed toxemia. I was a very weak and sick little boy. My wonderful parents did all they could for me and more; for this I will always be grateful. The policy in those days was to leave all smaller babies at hospital until they weighed at least six pounds (which in my case, took six weeks), so my mum would express milk every day and Dad would drive it to the hospital for me. When they took me home I was still so small Mum and Dad wrapped me in a shopping basket designed to carry two pounds of butter. I developed asthma and many other health problems and this continued until I changed my diet and lifestyle and cured myself in my mid-20s.

As a child and teenager I can clearly remember doctors telling me many times, 'You are an asthmatic and you will be for life. The best thing we can offer is medication. You just have bad genes. Keep taking the drugs.' I was given steroid injections, and a Ventolin inhaler and an Intal puffer, and told that I should take two puffs when I got an attack, every four hours as needed. One clever doctor told me not to drink cow's milk when I was having an attack. This was the only good advice I ever received. Years later, when learning about asthma, I discovered that the chest is one of the last parts of the human body that develops fully in the womb, during the eighth and ninth months, both of which I missed when I arrived into this world early. Funny that.

Still sick

At age 18, I woke up one morning, after one too many all-night drinking sessions with my two oldest friends Dave and Kerry, crawled out of bed and stumbled on to the bus to work. As the bus moved and swayed, I couldn't hold back. I vomited all over the bus floor, Kerry watching in hysterics. This was a low point for me. That day, I realised that I actually never enjoyed the drinking. It made me bloated, and I always suffered badly the next day. I was drinking and doing drugs (dope) because everyone else was. I was an insecure 'sheeple.' I gave up drink and drugs on the spot. It's one one of the best decisions I have ever made.

Three years later I was still getting colds, flu and coughs every year. I would be in bed for up to a week at a time, coughing, nose dribbling and feeling foul all over. I also had long-term lower back pain, which used to throb and would leave me in tears because of the long, deep aching that went on and on. It was always in the background, even when the acute pain died down.

Asthma is as scary as hell

I was still a bad asthmatic. Asthma is the most frightening and debilitating thing that I have ever experienced. Generally, whenever you hurt yourself or you are in pain, you know that you will be okay. However, asthma attacks you at the core as it is your breath that is taken away.

I couldn't count the times that, in the middle of the night, I would cry in despair, praying for sleep, but I was unable to lie down for fear of not breathing and dying. Panic would set in and the overwhelming fear was that I might die if I didn't get any more air into my lungs.

When you lose your breath, the best thing to do is to calm down and relax, but of course when you can't seem to get enough air, the opposite happens. You become stressed and upset and sometimes, particularly in children, you start to cry, which limits your air intake even further.

It is a devastating, terrifying and humbling experience. I genuinely thought I might die many, many times during those long dark nights of breathlessness. All my concentration was focused on getting air into my lungs; just breathing, just breathing, just breathing …

Hitting a crossroads

The asthma was stifling my life and stopping me from living fully in so many ways. I was taking 16 shots of Ventolin most days for many years. I had also developed bad skin and had pimples and bumps all over my face and body, with seemingly no rhyme nor reason. No amount of medical potions or creams ever worked to get rid of them. To add to all this I suffered from bad hayfever, oily skin, poor digestion, bloating, long-term constipation, fatigue, tiredness, and I was overweight. At one stage my weight got up to 80 kg, chubby for a man of my stature (I now weigh a lean and healthy 70 kg, as I did when I was a teenager).

To be blunt, I was a mess. My girlfriend at the time was studying to become a naturopath (a natural medical practitioner). She looked me in the face one day in a moment of brutal honesty and said, 'You are pathetic. You take drugs all the time for your sickness and yet you do nothing about it. Why don't you try something different? Take some responsibility; change your life and stop eating all that crap food. You are not going to be an effective father if you are sick all the time. Stop the complaining and the drug taking and get to the real cause of the problems instead: your diet.'

What? I thought my sickness was just 'genetics' or 'bad luck'?

As you can imagine, I was highly insulted and took this rather badly and personally. There was no connection between my diet and my sickness! Or any illness for that matter! At least, no one had ever told me that before. I thought that food was just fuel for the body (the TV adverts had always told me to 'eat meat for iron and protein' and to 'drink cow's milk every day to get strong bones'). And yet, after sitting on my bed sulking in the darkness for a few hours, I got over myself and realised something.

I did want to cure my asthma and my health problems. I did want more energy, vitality and strength. I wanted to feel young, alive and 100% free of illness. I wanted to be fit, healthy, and energetic. I wanted to be free from pain, to feel happy and to be able to breathe and run around with my kids until they were old enough to have their own kids. And then some.

I wanted a better life and I wanted to be in Full. Control. Of. It.

I wanted to rid myself of the sickness that was dominating my life.

The 'aha' moment

It dawned on me that as much as I hadn't enjoyed it, what my girlfriend had pointed out was quite simply the truth. I knew nothing about the link between food and illness. This was a powerful turning point for me. I had to admit that I had no idea of what to do and that the medical establishment I had been relying on for years could not help me. I had to open my mind to different ways of thinking. Up until then I had been doing nothing. I had ceded my power and personal responsibility to doctors who told me I was 'incurable' and it was just 'bad luck in the gene pool'. I realised that I had to ask for help in different places and I had to start 'unlearning all that I had learnt,' as the great Yoda said.

The best fruit is always the hardest to pick, so I took responsibility for my health and opened my mind to new ideas. I became focused on curing my body of all illness. I was willing to do whatever it took. Initially, the questions I started asking and the answers I got went against my thinking in so many ways. I had been told that my genes were prone to asthma and disease and that all I could do was take the medicine prescribed. This, I learned, is called 'The Local Theory of Disease'.

This theory suggests that illness is caused by a single agent acting at a single site in the body (then you treat the single agent with drugs). The very first new thing I discovered was a completely different and more holistic view called 'The Constitutional Nature of Disease'. This theory maintains that illness and disease are the result of multiple systems throughout the body breaking down. I was inspired by the notion that if I followed this line of thinking it meant I could potentially rebuild my body from scratch and cure my illnesses; something I have subsequently achieved.

Asking for help

I went to a naturopath who suggested swimming, as it was good for training the breathing process. Swimming was very helpful. I also read Louise Hay's book *You Can Heal Your Life*. Louise wrote that the asthma colour was yellow, so I dyed all my clothes and shoes yellow and wore only yellow for six months. Did wearing yellow help? I have no idea, but it certainly made lots of people laugh (particularly my bestest ever friend Robert) at my bad-taste yellow outfits, which is a good thing I guess ...

The point I make here is that I was willing to change, willing to do the work to get well, and willing to admit I knew NOTHING about what was required to make and maintain these changes. I had zero knowledge about nutrition or how the body worked.

However, I didn't care about what I had to do, just as long as I got to reclaim my health and my life.

Study, learn, research, CHANGE

I studied. I studied hard. Food, diet, fasting, exercise, flexibility, calories, acid versus alkaline, vitamins, minerals, antioxidants, how the body works, traditional diets, the bowels, vegetables, fruits, wholegrains, meat and dairy products, the internal organs, intolerances, food ingredients, additives … the list went on and on. What became very clear to me was that if I really wanted to get well, to get to a level of super-health, then I was going to have to change my *behaviour*.

One of the hardest things for a human being to do is to change and then remain consistent with that change. Change does not always happen as we envision it, and it can be very hard to adjust to it. The big shift in thinking for me came when I realised that the pain of remaining the same was greater than the pain of changing.

The pain of having no energy, no breath, regular back pain, cold sores, constipation and bad skin was bad enough for me to change my life. Change, I discovered, was internal.

I was learning at an astronomical rate and I slowly started making progress with my health. Step by step, I learned little gems that gave me instant benefits. I went to seminars. I asked healthy people for advice about what they did. I tried different eating regimes such as macrobiotic, vegan, fasting, raw foods and elimination diets, and I found golden rules in each. I devoured books. Over six years, a miracle happened. I cured my body and totally transformed my health and my life. Was it easy? No, it wasn't, but it was worth it.

Before you read any further, please note:

1. I advocate total self-responsibility when it comes to your health.

2. You may have to consider a different point of view for the advice in this book to work for you. Try to remain open.

3. The advice in this book is based on centuries of evidence of what seems to work best for most human beings, regardless of race, faith, creed, blood type, body type, size, constitutional type or genotype.

4. I suggest some things that may seem controversial or downright loopy. I suggest them because my experience to date has shown they work and I trust and believe they do.

5. Some ideas you currently think or believe are 'the truth' about food or your health may not actually be true at all.

6. Getting well, for most people, will take at least 12 months of hard work.

This book is for anyone interested in better health

The advice in this book has evolved by following and learning from the oldest and healthiest peoples on earth. How do they live to become healthy, drug-free and disease-free centenarians? What can they can teach us?

Their advice usually means a lifestyle change. Think of it like changing jobs; you learn different skills in new areas that literally change your experience of life.

The word 'diet' is from the Greek word 'diaita', meaning 'lifestyle', and that is what this book is all about – changing to an enjoyable, appetising, varied, healthy lifestyle that promotes and supports longevity. There is no specific religious or spiritual base to this book. It is for everyone. However, a positive attitude is important. Thoughts begin and then action follows, so if you read this book from the positive perspective of 'what can I learn here?', then you will discover pure health-gold in these pages. Using a positive approach, it is most likely you will transform your health.

Real health is all but forgotten by most people

Health is much more than the absence of disease. Real health is where the mind and body are functioning at peak efficiency and strength. Right now people everywhere are getting sicker, not healthier. I have known people in their 30s and 40s who have suffered or died from osteoporosis, Irritable Bowel Syndrome (IBS), asthma, obesity, diabetes, heart disease, stroke, stomach cancer, bone cancer, breast cancer, diverticulitis, depression, gout and arthritis. I have seen the devastation that occurs when someone dies young. And we think this is acceptable? We think that getting fat or obese, having rising blood pressure and cholesterol, losing our strength and libido, is just part of aging and is 'normal'? In the Western world it may be, but everywhere else it isn't. We consistently hear the message that we are 'living longer than ever', but this is simply not true.

As reported worldwide on 2 April 2013, the latest surveys show that health and longevity is the number one concern we have now.[1] Sadly, longevity increases are starting to slow across the Western world. Experts from Cardiff and Vale University Health Board,[2] the University of Calgary in Alberta in the *Canadian Journal of Cardiology*,[3] the Paris-based Organisation for Economic Co-operation and Development (OECD),[4] and The Institute for Health Metrics and Evaluation (IHME) at the University of Washington,[5] say the same thing. The pandemic of having a poor diet and being overweight or obese will significantly lower life expectancy for the next generation of children and young people.

What do I mean by this?

A major British study released in August 2013 is typical of what the next generation of children and young people are doing.

► 80% of 5–15-year olds are not eating five portions of fruit and vegetables daily.

► 50% of 5–15-year olds have chocolates or sweets daily.

► 40% of 13-year olds drink a soft drink every day.

► 25% of 5–15-year olds are inactive for 12 daytime hours in the weekend.

► 50% of 15-year olds go without breakfast.

► 70% of 13-year olds watch at least two hours of television on a weekday.[6]

The experts commented on this, and their warnings about the impact these behaviours will have on the future health, longevity, ability to work and possibility of a healthy aging process for these youngsters, were blunt. Simon Gillespie, Chief Executive of the British Heart Foundation, said, 'These figures are a warning that many of our children are in grave danger of developing coronary heart disease in the future if they continue to live the same lifestyle. I have seen some cases of high cholesterol in teenagers that you would expect to see in a stereotypical sedentary truck driver eating a cooked breakfast every day. We've got a generation growing up which will buck that trend and potentially they will be the generation that live less long than the generation above them. It really is as stark as that. If that isn't a wake-up call, then what is? Our expectations of what childhood is have to change. We almost have to reset what we regard as moderation – moderation is not cutting down from two burgers a day to one, it's cutting down to two burgers a week.'

Younger people who are obese do
have a higher risk of dying early.

Dr Katherine Flegal and colleagues at the
National Center for Health Statistics, USA, August 2013

In another American study, similar comments were forthcoming:

A 5-year-old growing up today is living in an environment where obesity is much more the norm than was the case for a 5-year-old a generation or two ago. Drink sizes are bigger, clothes are bigger and greater numbers of a child's peers are obese. And once someone is obese, it is very difficult to undo. So, it stands to reason that we won't see the worst of the epidemic until the current generation of children grows old.

Bruce Link, Professor of Epidemiology and Sociomedical Sciences at Columbia University's Mailman School of Public Health, New York City, August 2013

Existing literature largely indicates roughly about 5% of all adult deaths in the United States could be associated with overweight or obesity. What we find is that between the ages of 40 and 85 ... about 18% of all deaths that took place between 1986 and 2006 could be said to be associated with high body mass. The effects on obese children may be much worse. Obesity has dramatically worse health consequences than some recent reports have led us to believe. Previous research has likely underestimated obesity's impact on US mortality. Importantly, counter to most extant research, obesity's effect on mortality risk grows stronger with increasing age. From our findings, obesity actually has a very strong and substantial effect on old age mortality risk. We found that obesity indeed has a quite significant effect on mortality levels in the United States and estimates are actually significantly larger than prevailing wisdom has suggested. Successive cohorts are living in this new environment and are at greater risk of obesity at earlier times in their lives. Each specific cohort looks like a wave that's grown bigger than the cohort that has come before it. Adults born in the 1970s and 1980s – a generation for whom excess weight has been widespread and lifelong – will suffer higher premature death rates than have older Americans. We expect that obesity will be responsible for an increasing share of deaths in the United States and perhaps even lead to declines in US life expectancy. We believe we have a clearer picture of how obesity is impacting the [United States] population. Not only is the problem more serious than previously thought, it is destined to get worse as younger generations move into adulthood. It's quite worrisome. The absence of evidence of the obesity effect in older people is likely because obese people are more likely to experience early death, or they have serious health complications that would reduce their participation in health surveys. Barring any revolutionary breakthrough to lessen the prevalence, we're likely to see that obesity is going to account for a larger share [of deaths] in the future.

Ryan K. Masters, PhD, a Robert Wood Johnson Foundation Health and Society Scholar and Demographer at Columbia University's Mailman School of Public Health in New York City, and Associate Professor of Sociology at the University of Colorado at Boulder, Department of Sociology, USA, August 2013

What we are doing isn't working

For most of the 150,000 years of human evolution, we ate a fresh, local, balanced, plant-based wholefood diet. We were used to going without food for periods of time and eating raw or freshly caught provisions. Now we have too much food to eat, most of it highly processed and nutritionally empty. The top foods bought each week in most modern countries are now wine, beer, cow's milk, white sugar and sweeteners, white flour, processed cheese, white bread products, fizzy/soft/energy/soda/cola drinks, processed meats, coffee and takeaway foods. How is the state of our health as a result of consuming this food? Not well at all.

2

Non-communicable diseases: a global crisis?

Most people think we are living longer, healthier lives, when in fact longevity is declining. The next generation is predicted to live shorter lives than us, and people are getting far sicker, at much younger ages, all over the Western world.

Jason Shon Bennett

Observation

When studying something you must do a few things well. Observe, gather evidence, form a hypothesis, research your findings, look at history, follow a variety of human experience, double-check, and then use your common sense and intelligence. Then report.

This has been my objective while creating this book. Observation that is not led by emotion or money is the foundation of every science. Science is said to be a reporting of the truth for the wellbeing of humanity. However, you do not have to be a scientist to observe and draw conclusions.

In our health mentoring programme, 'thelifeplan®', I have observed hundreds of people. I have studied people who live long healthy lives without disease or drugs. I observed their habits, their commonalities, what they did, and what they didn't do. I have looked at large population groups (epidemiological studies), centenarians, traditional cultures, food habits, the Mediterranean diet, the Asian diet, the caveman diet, raw foods, the Paleolithic diet, fasting and more. I have looked at the science and the scientific research on people and how they live all over the world. This book represents the starting point of the conclusions I have reached through my study, observation and research.

An open and inquisitive mind?

I once had a conversation with an acquaintance at a dinner party who swore black and blue that she had an open mind. She said, 'I feed my kids red meat because without red meat you will die from a lack of iron.' When I quietly mentioned that I had raised my four children without red meat and that I personally had not eaten red meat for almost 30 years, she quickly changed the subject.

Iron is a great example of how so many people are influenced by marketing. You may have noticed the advertisements encouraging you to 'Eat your meat and get your iron'. This had led to a great number of us assuming that we need to eat meat to have good iron levels. I have not eaten meat for almost 30 years and my iron levels are very good. Whenever I go to donate blood the first thing the nurses do is prick my finger to check for quality. More often than not, they'll make a comment along the lines of, 'Goodness me, your blood is amazing – so high in iron and nutrients. Can we take a double amount? Have you just eaten a steak?' At this point I'll say, 'Sit down, we need to talk about where iron comes from.' Then I give them a lecture! Consider this: given that New Zealand women eat more red meat than almost any other group of women in the world, and health authorities regularly suggest that around 70% of New Zealand women are low in iron at any one time, how does eating meat fix your iron levels? A low iron level can be the result of a deficiency in one of several facets of what produces iron in our bodies. Eating meat is not a 'one-stop' solution.

In April 2014 our eldest son, Trey, turned 25. He is lean, vibrant, healthy and incredibly strong, and he has smashed a Guinness World Record; all without eating meat. The point here is that there are probably many things you believe about nutrition that may not be true, or as irrefutable as you think. They may in fact be completely bogus. Enough advertising can make you believe anything, true or false.

T. Colin Campbell, PhD, former Senior Science Advisor to the American Institute for Cancer Research, and Director of the Cornell-China-Oxford Project on Nutrition, Health and Environment 1983–1990, is the author of the comprehensive study on nutrition, *The China Study*. He sums up the tension between fact and fiction in his study, saying, 'Sustaining controversy as a means of discrediting findings that cause economic or social discomfort is one of the greatest sins in science.'

I agree with his words completely. If we find something uncomfortable then we do not talk about it; even if it is killing us and our children. You can attend a funeral and watch people smoke, drink copious amounts of alcohol and eat massive plates of constipating food while they mourn a friend or family member who died from a preventable modern disease.

Obesity and diabetes

In 1980, the biggest problem we had was global starvation, or 'not enough food.' Now, only 40 years on, we are dying of 'non-communicable diseases' (NCDs), almost all of which are preventable through diet and lifestyle changes.

Today, the biggest problem we have is obesity and too much of the wrong kinds of foods, alongside smoking, alcohol and poor lifestyle choices. We know that being overweight, obese or having type II diabetes is 99% preventable, yet we are suffering the biggest pandemic explosion of weight problems, obesity and diabetes in human history. During the last several decades there has been a systematic underestimation of the deadly hazards of obesity and being overweight, and how it causes early mortality, heart disease and cancers. Preventable lifestyle diseases such as obesity, cardiovascular disease and cancer now account for 70% of all global deaths.

A global picture

▶ 12% of the world's population is now obese.[1]

▶ 30% of all humans are now overweight.[2]

▶ Obesity rates have increased 82% worldwide in 20 years.[3]

▶ The dangerously overweight have doubled in number since 1980.[4]

▶ Every person in the world has gained more than 1 kilogram, on average, each decade since 1980.[5]

▶ By 2015, over two billion people will be obese (out of seven billion).[6]

▶ Obesity is now the number two cause of death, after tobacco. Obesity will soon overtake tobacco as the leading avoidable cause of premature death worldwide.[7]

> Obesity in NZ is a public health disaster ... It is a tragedy
> at the personal, family and social levels. It's a pandemic.
>
> Professor Robert Beaglehole, World Health Organisation (WHO)

► Numbers of overweight kids are growing by 1.3 million per year.[8]

► By 2020, 10% of the Western world could be suffering with diabetes; by 2010, 366 million people worldwide had diabetes.[9]

► In 1980, just 2% of all new type II diabetes cases were in children; by 2000, over 50% of all new diabetes cases were in children.[10]

► Unmanaged cases of diabetes are responsible for more than 50% of all heart attacks, 50% of strokes and 66% of all blindness.[11]

► The current generation of children and young people will be the first since 1960 to have higher mortality rates than their parents due to cardiovascular disease, stroke and far higher rates of type II diabetes.[12]

► Three times more people die now from 'overweight' than from 'malnutrition'.[13]

New Zealand

► Obesity now kills more New Zealanders than smoking.[14]

► 29% of New Zealanders are obese.[15]

► In some areas of New Zealand the obesity rate is 40%.[16]

► New Zealand adults are now the **second fattest** in the developed world.[17]

► There are 2.5 million overweight Kiwis, 1 million of them obese.[18]

► 31% of New Zealand children are now overweight before they hit puberty.[19]

► 27% of New Zealanders have diabetes or are at high risk of diabetes.[20]

► Diabetes is the number one initiating cause of New Zealand death, killing 4000 people each year.[21]

► 29% of New Zealanders will get cancer.[22]

Australia

► Obesity is now the number one cause of premature death in Australia.[23]

► By 2025 (just over ten years), there will be more obese Australians than healthy weight Australians.[24]

► Australian obesity is now at an all time high of 28%.[25]

► Female obesity has risen by 58% in ten years (2002–2012)[26] and female morbid obesity has risen by 70% in ten years.[27]

► Over 21% of Australian kids are overweight by age five.[28]

► Over 25% of teenagers are now obese.[29]

► Over 70% of Australian men are overweight or obese.[30]

► In 1998 there were 558 weight-loss surgeries performed in Australia. In 2010, 18,000 procedures were performed.[31]

► The top five causes of death in Australia now are poor diet, high blood pressure, smoking, being overweight and a lack of exercise.[32]

► Healthy life expectancy in Australia has reduced by about ten years.[33]

'... 736,000 more adult Australians are
now obese than in 2007 ...'

Roy Morgan Chief, Michele Levine, 2013

India

► India now has over 20% of its population overweight (from historically being the slimmest race in the world).[34]

► Diabetes will double (at least) to 70 million people within 20 years.[35]

► India lost 17.9 million healthy years due to NCDs in the last five years.[36]

China

► In 1982, 7% of the Chinese population was obese.[37] In 2002, 25% of Chinese adults were overweight or obese.[38]

► In 1985, 1% of boys were overweight.[39] Today, 35% of boys are overweight or obese.[40]

► In 2002, 25% of Chinese adults were overweight or obese.[41] Today, 40% of Chinese adults are overweight or obese.[42]

► There are 103 million Chinese with diabetes; that is, 1 in 10 adults.[43]

United States of America

▶ Obesity now kills 25% of Americans.[44]

▶ 36% are obese, more than one in three.[45]

▶ Obesity is predicted to affect 50–60% of Americans by 2030.[46]

> During the last several decades, there has been a systematic underestimation of the hazards of obesity. I am deeply concerned that the United States is the fattest society in the world and likely to be the fattest in the history of the world. Unfortunately, most people prefer prescription of pills to prescription of healthy lifestyles. The export of our diet and lifestyle, which increases rates of obesity, together with tobacco, to developing countries will result in cardiovascular disease emerging as the leading killer in the world.
>
> Dr Charles H. Hennekens, USA, February 2013

▶ Over 80% of men and 77% of women are overweight.[47]

▶ Being overweight is now considered 'normal'.[48]

▶ By 2020, 75% of American adults will likely be obese.[49]

▶ By 2048, every US adult will be overweight.[50]

▶ US children's obesity rates have increased 300% in 20 years.[51]

▶ The average American has gained 500 grams each year since 1995.

> In the wake of the obesity epidemic, we've got a diabetes epidemic. Diabetes is linked to our epidemic of obesity, and like obesity, it can be prevented. I expect it to continue to rise as long as obesity rates continue to rise.
>
> Thomas Farley, New York Health Commissioner, 2013.

> Fully one in eight adults – approximately 29 million people – now report that they have been diagnosed with type II diabetes.
>
> Humphrey Taylor, Harris Poll Chairman, USA, 2013

▶ 36% of the population is obese – more than one in three people.

- US baby boomers have 30% higher rates of obesity, 46% more diabetes, 38% more hypertension and 5.9-fold more hypercholesterolemia than their parents had at the same age.[52]

- One in eight Americans has been diagnosed with type II diabetes.[53]

- In northern America, a new diabetic is diagnosed every 40 seconds.[54]

- New York now has one diabetes death every 90 minutes, and rising.

- Over 80% of US adults of Pacific Island descent are overweight or obese.[55]

- 23% of 15-month-old American Samoan children are obese. This is the highest rate of child obesity in the world.[56]

Canada

- Over 60% of men are overweight or obese.[57]

- Obesity rates in Canada are now a record 25% and rising.[58]

- Canadian diabetics have a 51% higher risk of death than those without diabetes.[59]

Latin America

- Obesity is now growing fastest in Latin America.[60]

- 50% of Brazilians are now overweight and 15% are obese.[61]

Mexico[62]

- Diabetes is now the number one killer in Mexico.

- 38 new diabetes cases are diagnosed every hour (900 per day, 6000 per week).[63] Ten million Mexicans now have diabetes.

- Mexicans are now the number two most obese country behind the United States.

- Obesity levels have tripled in the past three decades.

- Mexico has the worst childhood obesity rates anywhere in the world; over 35% of children are obese.

- Over 82% of Mexican women are overweight or obese; there are 21 million clinically obese adults in Mexico.

- In 2000–2006, there were 270,000 diabetes deaths in Mexico; in 2006–2012, there were 482,654 diabetes deaths in Mexico. This is a 79% increase in six years.

- Ten million Mexicans now have diabetes.

Europe

- Obesity levels in the EU hit an all-time record high in 2013. 50% of all EU citizens are overweight or obese.[63]

- 40% of all EU children are obese.[64]

- In Hungary, Ireland and Malta every fourth citizen is seriously overweight.[65]

- 60% of men and 43% of women in Germany are overweight[66]

- Swedish diabetics aged 20–44 have a 70–80% higher risk of death than average.[67]

- In 2003, 18% of Turks, or 12.6 million people, were overweight; by 2012, 35% of Turks, or 25.9 million, were overweight.[68]

> The prevalence of overweight and obesity is now described as a global epidemic and major public health problem throughout Europe. Childhood obesity has reached epidemic proportions in Europe, with body weight now the most prevalent childhood disease.
>
> Dr Sinead Murphy, consultant paediatrician,
> Temple Street Hospital, Ireland, 2013

United Kingdom and Ireland

- Over 30% of UK children are overweight or obese by the age of nine;[69] the UK has the highest rate of child obesity in Western Europe.[70]

- In the ten years 2001–2011, UK childhood obesity rates grew by 300%.[71]

- By 2020, 80% of UK men and 70% of UK women will be overweight.[72]

- One in ten British children aged 4–5 years is now obese.[73]

- Overweight and obese UK adults increased from 58% to 65% of the population in men and from 49% to 58% in women from 1993–2011.[74]

▶ British obesity has grown 50% in six years from 2005–2011.[75]

▶ Obese UK adults went from 13% in 1993 to 24% in 2011 for men, and from 16% to 26% for women.

▶ UK diagnosis of obesity in NHS hospitals was 1019 in 2002. UK diagnosis of obesity in NHS hospitals was 11,736 in 2012. This is 11 times higher in just a decade.[76]

▶ Scottish obesity rates are 27% and climbing.[77]

▶ Scottish obesity-related deaths have risen by 20% in just five years (2007–2012).[78]

▶ Scottish obesity in boys age 2–4 has grown 60% in the last two years,[79] and 15% of Scottish children are now obese before they get to school.[80]

▶ 25% of Irish primary school children are now overweight or obese.[81]

▶ UK diabetes rates (age 1–40) are now six times higher than in the 1990s.[82]

▶ One in eight UK people diagnosed with diabetes is now under 40 years of age. Twenty years ago, it was one in 30.[83]

▶ Diabetes UK expects the number of people in Britain with diabetes to rise by 700,000 by 2020. This forecasts 4.4 million people in the UK alone will have diabetes by 2020.[84]

▶ UK diabetics have a 65% higher risk of death than non-diabetics.

▶ 160,000 Welsh (5% of the population) have now been diagnosed in a diabetes epidemic that continues to grow, with 350,000 more people medically diagnosed as pre-diabetic.[85]

▶ The number of UK children on obesity drugs grew 1500% in just seven years (1999–2006), and it is still rising.[86]

Not only is the number of people dying from obesity rising, but more toddlers than ever are being registered obese. What more warning could we possibly need that this crisis has to be addressed? And it has to be addressed at once.

Jackson Carlaw, Health Spokesman,
UK, June 2013

> The younger you get diabetes, the worse your outlook and the more 'life years' you lose. It is the younger people who have the most risk of dying. That is quite frightening considering the number of people being diagnosed at a younger age.
>
> Professor Tony Barnett, University of Birmingham,
> UK, June 2013

France

▶ Obesity rates have doubled in 15 years over the period 1997–2012, to reach seven million.[87]

▶ 15% of the French population is now obese; 41% of the population is now overweight.[88]

▶ French obesity levels for ages 18–24 have grown by 35% in three years (2006–2009).[89]

Middle East

▶ Diabetes rates in the Middle East will double (at least) within 15 years.[90]

▶ 40% of Saudis are obese and 20,000 Saudis die every year due to obesity.[91]

▶ Over 80% of Saudi children are obese.[92]

▶ Over 20% of Israeli teenagers are overweight.[93]

Heart disease

A global picture

▶ Heart disease, cardiovascular disease (CVD) and high blood pressure (hypertension) are 95% preventable.

▶ In 1920, American physician Sir William Osler wrote, 'You could expect to see one patient per hospital suffering from heart problems.'

▶ From 1920–1930, cardiologist Dr Paul White spent ten years searching England for anyone with heart disease; he found three cases. A hundred years later, heart disease is the number one killer worldwide.[94]

▶ Heart disease kills 30% of all humans, that's 17 million deaths each year.[95]

▶ In 1913, the average 40+ man had a 1% chance of a heart attack before age 65;[96] in 2013, the average 40+ man has a 50% chance of a heart attack before 65.[97]

▶ Heart disease is the number one killer of women, causing one in three female deaths. This is about one death per minute.[98]

▶ Heart failure is set to rise 46% in the next 15 years in the US.[99]

▶ High blood pressure is a major cause of death worldwide, killing over nine million people every year.[100]

▶ Almost 78 million adults have high blood pressure, which is now the biggest global risk factor for disease and early death.[101]

▶ In 1990 the most deaths were caused by malnutrition (not enough food). A mere 30 years later, most deaths are caused by high blood pressure (too much bad food).[102]

▶ The WHO estimates that the number of people who will die from heart disease will be over 23 million per year by 2030.[103]

▶ Heart disease now kills 9600 Chinese every day. This is around one Chinese person every ten seconds.[104]

New Zealand[105]

▶ A New Zealander now dies every 90 minutes from heart disease.

▶ Heart disease kills 40% of all Kiwis.

▶ Heart disease kills four times more women than breast cancer.

▶ New Zealand has the second highest stroke rate in the modern world.

We know that the longer you're overweight, the higher
the risk of cardiovascular disease in adult life.
Professor Barry Taylor, University of Otago, NZ

Australia

▶ Over 30% of Australians have high cholesterol yet only 10% of them are aware they have the condition.[106]

India and Pakistan

► 25% of heart disease victims in India are aged under 40.[107]

► Up to 90,000 Indian children are getting heart ailments every year.[108]

► Ischaemic heart disease is India's number one cause of death.[109]

► 35% of all deaths in Pakistan are caused by CVD.[110]

► India is set to witness a spike in deaths due to heart diseases, far exceeding that of China.[111]

► In 2004, 14% of total deaths in India were due to heart disease; by 2030, this is expected to more than double.[112]

United States of America

► Every day, 2000 Americans die from CVD.[113]

► Heart failure is the number one cause of hospitalisation for Americans over 65.[114]

► There are 900,000 heart attacks annually.[115]

► 600,000 people die from CVD every year; that is one death every 40 seconds.[116]

► Heart disease will affect 50% of all Americans.[117]

► 45-year-old US men have a 60% lifetime chance of heart disease; 45-year-old US women have a 55% lifetime chance of heart disease.[118]

> Heart disease is a food-borne illness. 99% of heart disease
> is preventable by changing your diet and lifestyle.
>
> Dr Dean Ornish, Clinical Professor of Medicine,
> University of California, USA

Europe[119]

► Heart disease is the number one killer in Europe.

► Heart disease causes 40% of all deaths in Europe.

► CVD accounts for nearly two million EU deaths each year.

What is the worst thing about these preventable high blood pressure, heart disease, stroke and CVD deaths? In the USA, barely 3% of the healthcare budget for cardiovascular disease is spent on prevention, even though 95% of heart disease is preventable through changes in diet, lifestyle and exercise.

Cancer

A global picture

▶ Almost 70% of all new cancer cases each year are preventable and related solely to smoking, alcohol, weight, exercise or a poor diet. Over 95% of cancers are preventable; only 5% are strongly hereditary or genetic.[120]

▶ In 1900, cancer was a rare disease, causing just 1% of deaths. In 1913, Frederick L. Hoffman started the American Cancer Society (ACS) stating 'diet was the way to prevent and treat cancer'.

▶ In the 1970s, the 70-page 'Cancer Review' from the International War on Cancer said, 'genetics determines about 2–3% of total cancer risk'.

▶ Cancer is growing in more than half of all countries worldwide in 2013.[121]

▶ Cancer is the second most common cause of death worldwide, killing 7.6 million people per year and rising; it now kills one in eight people worldwide (more than Aids, malaria and tuberculosis combined).[122]

▶ Cancer kills more than 25% of people in Western countries.[123]

▶ Since 1980, obesity and cancer rates have doubled.[124]

▶ Men now have three times the cancer rate of their grandfathers. Prostate cancer rates have risen 500% since 1980.[125]

▶ There are 1 million new cases of stomach cancer each year.[126]

▶ Cancer is increasing by 15% every year,[127] and global cancer cases are projected to rise by another 75% by 2030.[128]

Cancer, alcohol and tobacco

▶ Over 30% of cancer deaths are due to tobacco use.[129]

▶ Smokers are 23 times more likely to develop lung cancer.[130]

▶ Alcohol accounts for 5% of all cancer deaths.[131]

▶ Alcohol raises the risk of liver, breast, colon, mouth, esophagus, larynx and pharynx cancers.[132]

> The genes have been there for thousands of years,
> but if cancer rates are changing in a lifetime,
> that doesn't have much to do with genes.
>
> Dr Michelle Holmes, Cancer Specialist from
> Harvard University, USA

New Zealand

► Cancer now causes 29% of all New Zealand deaths, killing 8000 people every year.[133]

► New Zealand women have the highest rate of bowel cancer in the world.[134]

► New Zealand men have the third highest rate of bowel cancer in the world.[135]

► Bowel cancer is 97% preventable as it is only 3% genetic.[136]

Australia

► Cancer is the number two killer in Australia, now causing over 30% of all deaths.[137]

China[138]

► There is a new cancer case diagnosed in China every ten seconds.

► There are now two million cancer deaths every year and rising in China.

► Over 50% of all adult men smoke; over 40% of Chinese doctors smoke.

► The mortality rate from lung cancer has risen 465% in the last 30 years.

► Preventable lifestyle cancers of the lung, stomach, rectum, liver, and oesophagus are the most common in China. The age of Chinese cancer patients is now younger than ever before.

United States of America[139]

► The 2010 President's Cancer Panel expects 41% of Americans will get cancer.

► Over 1.6 million Americans get cancer every year.

► Every 12 months more Americans die of cancer than have died from all the wars the United States has ever fought combined.

▶ Even after adjusting for age, the 'War on Cancer' has not improved the percentage of Americans dying of cancer. The only improvement has been detection, not improving survival.

> The rise in cancer prevalence is tied to tobacco use, obesity, diet and a lack of physical activity. Half of cancer deaths are related to these preventable causes. Modifying personal behaviors to adopt a healthier lifestyle that eliminates or reduces these risks, where possible, could therefore, have a remarkable impact on our nation's burden of cancer.
>
> The number of cancer sufferers is expected to increase from 12 million in 2008 to 22 million in 2030.[140]

United Kingdom

▶ UK cancer incidence has increased by 35% in the past 20 years.[141]

▶ One in five UK cases of breast cancer is now in women under the age of 50.[142]

▶ In 2001, 33% of Britons who died had cancer; by 2008, 42% of Britons who died had cancer; by 2020, 50% of Britons who die will be diagnosed with cancer.[143]

▶ By 2030, cancer rates in Northern Ireland will have grown by 80%.[144]

Over 95% of people in the West now die from obesity, diabetes, cancer, heart disease, stroke, autoimmune diseases or smoking. Do you eat the typical modern daily diet? Around 3500 calories of nutrient poor, low fibre, sugar-rich refined carbohydrates, highly processed animal foods and toxic, rancid fats? If so, then your odds are 99 out of 100 to be included in one of the above statistics in your 60s or 70s after a long, slow and painful decline in health.

What are the world experts saying?

What do the world's best cardiologists, doctors, surgeons, health researchers, professors, epidemiologists, universities and scientists say?

We are giving incomplete risk information. The majority of adults who are considered to be at low risk for cardiovascular disease are actually at high risk across their remaining lifespan.

Donald Lloyd-Jones, Associate Professor, Northwestern University Feinberg School of Medicine, Chicago, USA

This generation of children may be the first that won't live as long as their parents ... they will live 2–5 years less.

The New England Journal of Medicine, USA, February, 2010

We are living sicker from preventable illnesses. Nearly a third of the US population (31%) have diagnosed high blood pressure, 9.5% have diabetes, and 27.8% are obese.

Dr Reed Tuckson, Executive Vice President and Chief of Medical Affairs of United Health Group, commenting on the 2012 'America's Health Rankings Report', USA

It is likely that in a few years we will see a similar epidemic of cardiovascular disease and, after that, probably an increase in a good number of cancers as well.

Professor Jason Halford, UK Association for the Study of Obesity, UK, 2013

There will be a generation of children who will die before their parents; they will develop diabetes, cancer, heart disease ...

Cardiff and Vale University Health Board, Wales, February, 2012

Sugar consumption is fueling the global epidemic of diabetes.

Dr Walter Willett, nutritionist and epidemiologist at the Harvard School of Public Health, USA

For most heart attack victims, diet alone would work if we advocated diet, but we don't.

Dr William P. Castelli, Medical Director of the Framingham Heart Study, USA, 1984

A vegetarian diet can prevent 97% of our coronary occlusions.

An American Medical Association editorial, 1961

... the next generation will live a shorter life span; it will be the first decline in life span since industrialization.

Norm R.C. Campbell, MD, University of Calgary in Alberta; Canada, February 2012

People are not really aware of what normal weight is any more. If you have got 70% of people overweight or obese, that has become normal viewing these days, not only for children but for parents as well.

Heather Yeatman, Public Health Association of Australia President, Australia, 2013

Thousands of cases of cancer could be prevented by maintaining a healthy weight, being regularly physically active and eating a plant-based diet without too much salt, alcohol or red and processed meat.

Dr Rachel Thompson, World Cancer Research Fund, UK, 2011

Not only is the number of people dying from obesity rising, but more toddlers than ever are obese. What more warning could we possibly need that this crisis has to be addressed? And it has to be addressed at once.

Jackson Carlaw, UK Health Spokesman, UK, June 2013

If the doctors of today will not become the nutritionists of tomorrow, the nutritionists of today will become the doctors of tomorrow.

Paavo O. Airola, Naturpathic Doctor, PhD, Canada

3

Advertising, marketing and medicine

Change is not something many of us like. We like things to remain as they are. However, change is inevitable and, indeed, is the one constant and reliable thing we have in our lives. When you embrace it, miracles can happen ...

Jason Shon Bennett

Advertising is designed to sell you stuff you don't need

Advertisers know that if you tell the subconscious mind something enough (usually around two dozen times), then it will believe it. This is why advertisers talk about 'frequency'. They need their adverts in front of you, telling you their story, over and over again, until your subconscious mind believes it. We are all 'marketed to' via the media every day. If you hear a message often enough your subconscious will believe it, even if it is completely untrue. A friend working in the food industry once said to me, 'But if it is on TV then it must be true, otherwise the broadcasting standards authority would step in!' Not at all. The food industry is one of the most powerful industries on earth.[1]

> Being healthy of body and mind right now is like
> a modern version of civil disobedience.
>
> Richard Linklater, filmmaker, USA

The television claims of 'healthy food' are generally bogus

Almost all television advertisements that contain nutritional claims for food promote junk food.[2] An in-depth Australian study proved this yet again in 2008.[3] The NSW Centre for Overweight and Obesity studied 714 hours of Sydney television broadcasts and found the unhealthy foods most advertised with emphasis on their 'nutritional value' were high sugar, low fibre breakfast cereals, cakes, muffins, biscuits, pies, battered meat and fast foods.

High fibre claims were made for low fibre, high sugar cereals. Reduced fat claims were made for high sugar cakes and biscuits. Low sugar, reduced fat and reduced energy content were the most common claims for chocolate, lollies, sweets and candies. This has been tested and proven by consumer groups all over the world. The majority of television food adverts aimed at children promote nutritionally void, unhealthy and constipating, acidic junk food![4]

This type of advertising is not marketing; it is lying and it is corrupt. One example is a well-known brand of cornflakes and coco pops. Both contain more sugar per gram than Coca Cola and more salt than a packet of potato chips.

These are heavily advertised foods promoted as breakfast cereals. Would you give your kids Coke and chips for breakfast?

> He who does not know food; how can he
> understand the diseases of man?
>
> Hippocrates

Some prevalent food myths

► By 1753, the consumption of fresh fruit, in particular limes, was known to cure scurvy. This information was ignored and countless thousands died of a preventable disease.

► Toxic mercury, which we now know causes cancer, was used as medicine in the 1900s.

► In the early 1900s, the original Coca Cola drink contained tiny amounts of cocaine and claimed to 'cure morphine addiction and impotence'.

- In the 1930s, doctors promoted a huge breakfast of fried, processed bacon and eggs as essential and healthy.

- In the 1940s, doctors believed that heart disease was merely the body getting worn out and said that diet couldn't possibly affect heart disease, as there was nothing people could do about it.

- DDT (Dichlorodiphenyltrichloroethane) was 'fine'. It has been discovered to cause chemical feminisation. In 1947, *Time* magazine ran an advert that said, 'DDT is good for me-e-e!' The accompanying text said, 'The great expectations held for DDT have been realized. During 1946, exhaustive scientific tests have shown that when properly used, DDT kills a host of destructive pests and it is a benefactor of all humanity.'

- In the 1950s, doctors promoted cigarettes as 'heart warming' and they were sold as a health product to 'ward off coughs and colds'. Doctors talked about which brand of cigarettes had the greatest health benefits, and many openly endorsed smoking in advertisements. Cigarette companies produced 'scientific studies' to prove how beneficial and healthy smoking was for the eyes, throat and chest.

- In the 1960s, food companies said many chemicals that were added to bread were 'harmless', until they were proven to be cancer causing and were banned.

- In the 1970s, sugar was marketed and sold as 'the magical healthful ingredient' you should 'add to everything!'

- During the 1970s scientists gave assurances that thalidomide was 'harmless'. It was, of course, discovered as the cause of hideous disfigurements.

- PCB chemicals were once used in appliances, fluorescent lighting, insulation and insecticides to name a few products. They were banned in the 1970s after being linked to higher cancer rates, type II diabetes and slow growth rates.

- Dioxin (possibly the most deadly chemical ever) was 'safe' in the herbicide 245-T.

- As recently as the 1980s, doctors in the United Kingdom and new Zealand would still advise pregnant women to, 'Go to the pub and have a drink,' to defer labour.[5]

► During the 1980s, drug companies made billions selling antacids for stomach ulcers, even when they knew ulcers were a bacterial problem that their product could not treat or cure.

► In the 1990s and 2000s, plastic industry spokesmen denied that the chemical bisphenol-A (BPA) was dangerous. BPA is a highly toxic endocrine disruptor linked to reproductive damage, cardiovascular disease, liver problems and diabetes. It is especially harmful for babies and children.

► In the 2000s, the food industry said that margarine was 'healthy' and 'lowered cholesterol'. They tried desperately to silence Dr Johanna Budwig, who exposed trans-fats laden margarine for what it is: a cheap, plastic product that causes cancers, diabetes, obesity and heart disease being sold as a 'health food'.

My point here is to be wary. The food and medicine industries have forgotten about health and have become dominated by the need to make more and more and more money.

> Modern medicine **can** manage trauma better than any other system of medicine; diagnose and treat many medical and surgical emergencies; treat acute bacterial infections with modern antibiotics; treat some parasitic and fungal infections; prevent many infectious diseases by immunization; diagnose complex medical problems; replace damaged hips and knees; get good results with cosmetic and reconstructive surgery; and it can diagnose and correct hormonal deficiencies.
>
> Modern medicine **cannot** treat viral infections; cure most chronic degenerative diseases; effectively manage most kinds of mental illness; cure most forms of allergy or autoimmune disease; effectively manage psychosomatic illnesses, or cure most forms of cancer.
>
> Dr Andrew Weil, MD, *Spontaneous Healing*, USA, 1995

For many the drugs don't work

Doctors are brilliant at prescribing drugs for pain relief, emergency healthcare and trauma; no doubt about it. If I broke my arm I would be running for the pain relief and the expertise they offer! However, preventative health and nutrition is not their area of expertise and many general practioners have not been taught or are not aware of the effectiveness of this approach. Hippocrates said, 'First, do no harm.' Most people believe drugs will cure a problem. Drugs can alleviate or mask symptoms, but they do little to alter the fundamental underlying health problem, which in most cases will continue, as does the patient's deterioration in health. A surgeon once said to me that we need 'conceptual adequacy' (I interpret this to mean a complete and thorough overview and understanding about a topic) to understand how different parts of the body works.

Symptoms are clues

The word 'symptom' is derived from the word 'signal'. Our symptoms are just that: signals from the body that something is not right. If the oil gauge light comes on in your car you can stop the signal (or symptom) by unscrewing the lightbulb. The signal goes away and presto, you have fixed the dying handbrake. Or have you? The car will run for a while but the underlying problem is not solved, cured or fixed. The next time you get a signal or symptom (in this case, brake failure), you may have a serious accident. The human body is the same. Health symptoms are the body telling you that something is wrong. You can either deal with it now, or deal with a much bigger and more deadly problem later. This is called living in a state of 'pre-illness'. Remember, doctors are not trained or paid to **prevent** disease, they are trained and paid to **treat** disease with drugs.

> As a doctor I was still getting a lot of questions about food and diet. One day I mentioned this uncomfortable situation to another young doctor. 'Just consult the dietitians if you have a problem,' she said after listening to my confession. 'They'll take care of it.' She paused for a moment, looked suspiciously around the nursing station, then leaned over and whispered, 'I know we're supposed to know about nutrition and diet, but none of us really does.' She was right. Nearly 20 years later, she may still be.
>
> A medical doctor commenting to *The New York Times*, 16 September 2010[6]

Medical schools don't teach the food → disease link

The reality is that most doctors have little idea about what foods to recommend that will transform your health or will prevent disease, because they are not trained in nutrition and food. Even though 90% plus of all modern diseases[7] are directly related to diet and lifestyle, medical school training focuses largely on drugs and surgical procedures. Some medical schools include no tuition about nutrition in their courses, focusing largely on disease, surgery and drug therapy (pharmacology).

> Within 15 years of completing my six-year degree, half of what
> I had learnt would be out of date. During my years of training
> I was required to attend just one class on nutrition.
>
> Dr Michael Mosley, *Sydney Morning Herald*, 20 September 2013.

'Doctore' means 'to teach' or 'to heal'

The Latin word 'doctore' means 'to teach' or 'to heal', not 'to promote drugs'. In the 1980s, the National Academy of Sciences published a report showing almost no adequate food and nutrition education in medical schools. In 2013, over 30 years later, nothing has changed. In fact, it has gotten worse, with the vast majority of medical schools failing to meet even the minimum recommended 25 hours of instruction.[8] In October 2013, I presented a seminar to a full house in Queenstown. In the audience was a doctor who, after the seminar, waited over an hour to talk with me. She said, 'I just loved what you had to say about diet and lifestyle changes and I will be sending my patients to you for food advice. In seven years of medical training to become a doctor, we had less than a day spent learning nutrition, so we really don't know anything about it at all. I also love how you work alongside doctors, and not in competition with them, as this is the future of healthcare.'

The nutrition training received by the average doctor during medical school is barely 2.5 hours. Doctors specialise in diagnosing ailments and disease. The basic medical training system is sponsored by the drug industry. Drugs are great at suppressing or hiding symptoms, but the biggest killers on Planet Earth are lifestyle diseases and **drugs do not cure lifestyle diseases**. Lifestyle diseases aren't infectious or invasive. You can't catch diabetes by not washing your hands. You can't kiss someone and catch cancer. You can't cure heart disease with a chemical or drug. These health issues are not contagious, spread by touch or wiped out by antibiotics.

Currently, the top causes of death in New Zealand are heart disease, strokes, cancer, obesity, autoimmune diseases and diabetes. Chronic degenerative diseases like these are latent, building for years before symptoms appear. They exist and are growing in the body well before there is an awareness of them. This is what I mean by being 'pre-ill'. Prevention is the cure and the cure is prevention. As the old saying goes, 'It's better to have a fence at the top of a cliff than an ambulance at the bottom.'

> Some physicians I have met refuse to accept the evidence that nutrition, exercise and lifestyle are our main defenses against disease. From the look of them, I suspect they do so because they want everyone to be condemned to the same mediocre health they suffer themselves.
>
> Dr Michael Colgan, Continuing Medical Education lectures, USA, 1992

Doctors have a very low life expentancy

It is ironic that doctors have a very low life expectancy, dying on average between the ages of 58 and 70, depending on the country. In 2011, at a pharmacy conference, an older doctor took me aside and cautioned me: 'Be careful, doctors hate change.' I know dieticians, chemists, pharmacists, doctors, naturopaths and nutritionists who are obese, sick, and unfit; they smoke and drink to excess and come to me for advice because they are unhappy with their health. I have worked with doctors from Scotland, the United Kingdom and the United States who have shown great interest in learning more about how to eat and live well.

One 2011 survey showed the probability that a healthy weight doctor would record an obesity diagnosis for an obese patient was 93%, while for overweight or obese doctors, it was just 7%.[9] So, if your doctor is overweight, they probably won't tell you that you are overweight, or that being overweight and obese is now one of the top two preventable causes of premature death in the world. Obesity is also higher in nurses.[10]

Doctors, alcohol abuse, depression and suicide

Heavy drinking among medical students is legendary. Studies have shown doctors are three times more likely than average to die as a result of alcohol-related cirrhosis of the liver. In Britain alone, more than 15,000 doctors suffer from drink and drug addictions.[11] That's one in six doctors. Depression among doctors is also much higher than average. Doctors have high levels of suicide, which have been attributed to a feeling that they 'need to have all the answers'.[12] Most doctors appear to give personal nutritional education a low priority too, with 40% of doctors experiencing burnout or work/life balance issues.[13] However, we go to them for longevity and life/health balance advice? Around 50% of male doctors in China smoke, and people go to them for health advice?

Remember, most doctors are amazing people!

Most of the doctors I have met are great people who are 100% committed to their patients and do a great and often life-saving job. However, there are two kinds of doctors: doctors who promote drugs, and doctors who want to get you well by whatever means possible. These doctors use a holistic approach to treatment and understand that lifestyle and diet are also essential for your long-term health. If your doctor scoffs at diet and wants you only to take drugs, simply change your doctor.

Find a great doctor who will listen to you; one who wants to get you well again by any means necessary, including using smart dietary and lifestyle changes.

> I just lectured 600 doctors at Kaiser. They are all fat.
>
> Dr Walter Bortz, Stanford University gerontologist, 2010,
> Boston Marathon runner, USA[14]

An unhealthy merger: the medical industry and the drug industry

Doctors and scientists have a hard time admitting diet and lifestyle are the keys to wiping out disease and increasing longevity. Breast cancer is a good example when considering this connection. When questioned about breast cancer and diet, many doctors maintain there is little evidence that diet has an effect on breast cancer and that as long as the patient is having treatment, the patient can eat whatever she or he likes. However, there is robust and undeniable evidence from hundreds of studies on millions of women all over the world proving that less than 10% of breast cancer is genetic.[15] Many mainstream cancer organisations have finally accepted and confirmed that most breast cancer is caused by poor diet and lifestyle choices. Even with this overwhelming evidence, some doctors and scientists maintain that it is unscientific to suggest that a body that is well fed is more able to resist disease than a poorly fed body.

'Dirty infected hands are fine while dealing with infectious diseases'

In the 1800s, Austrian Dr Ignaz Semmelweiss advocated hand washing among patients to keep hospitals clean and hygienic. He was branded a disgrace by the medical profession. A large number of surgeries were complicated by infection, there was a high risk of death due to poor hygiene practices, and hospitals earned a reputation as death houses. However, once hand washing was widely accepted, death rates for infectious diseases in hospital wards dropped by 90%. Initially, though, this radical idea was greeted with scepticism, ridiculed for being extreme and ignored by most doctors of the day.

Is a plant-based wholefood diet the new hand washing?

The authors of many large and peer-reviewed meta-analysis study projects, covering millions of people studied from all across the world, have commented that 'eating far more plants and far less meat' is one of the key steps for health and longevity. The groups and the studies include the World Cancer Research Fund (WCRF), the International 2013 GBD Study, the 2010 Heart and Stroke Statistics report published by the American Heart Association (compiled by an international consortium of nearly 500 scientists from 187 countries), the Harvard School of Public Health, and the most comprehensive report ever issued on cancer: the 351-page World Cancer Report issued by the International Agency for Research on Cancer and the WHO.

> When these patients commit to plant-based nutrition, they can not only halt but they can arrest and on occasion there will be significant evidence of disease reversal. It's getting to the point where it will be unconscionable for patients with cardiovascular disease not to be informed that this option exists.
>
> Dr Caldwell B. Esselstyn, retired heart surgeon, Cleveland Clinic, Ohio, January 2013

> This research is staggering and shows clear evidence that regular meat consumption contributes substantially to premature death. By simply replacing meat with other foods, 10% of male deaths and 8% of female deaths could be prevented.
>
> Dr Frank Hu, Harvard School of Public Health, USA, commenting on the 28-year study covering 120,000 people, March 2013

The World Cancer Research Fund and the American Institute for Cancer Research had independent scientists at Imperial College in London review all the 1012 'cancer and diet' studies in the medical literature. This was the most comprehensive, evidence-based research on cancer and diet ever undertaken. Following that, another Independent Expert Panel reviewed the results and made judgements. What did they recommend? 'Consume a plant-based diet. On meat, the clear message that comes out of our report is that red and processed meat increases risk of bowel cancer and that people who want to reduce their risk should consider cutting down the amount they eat.' Teresa Nightingale, General Manager of WCRF said, 'Many people feel confused about cancer prevention because it can seem like a new study is published every week that suggests that a new substance either causes or prevents cancer. But this takes the latest scientific findings and adds them to the existing body of evidence in a way that ensures our advice takes the latest research into account. This means people can be confident that our recommendations are up-to-date as well as being the most evidence-based information on cancer prevention available anywhere in the world. This latest report shows that there is enough evidence to recommend that people can reduce their bowel cancer risk by consuming less red and processed meat and alcohol, having more foods containing fibre, and by maintaining a healthy weight and being regularly physically active. This report confirms that bowel cancer is one of the most preventable types of cancer and we estimate that about 43% of bowel cancers cases in the UK could be prevented through these sorts of changes. That is about 17,000 cases every year.'[16]

The combination of eating a plant-based wholefood diet, making lifestyle changes and regular fasting is the most powerful thing I have seen, witnessed, done, followed, experienced and been a part of – ever. There are studies going back 100 years involving millions of people from all over the world on this subject.

They all say the same thing. Eat better, eat less and change what you do every day. Simple, isn't it? Why are we not doing it? Simple changes will probably add a few decades of wonderful health and vitality to your life, and may just save your life. However, the process requires (wait for it, take a deep breath, hold on!): **change.**

Cancer should not be a death sentence anywhere in the world as there are proven ways to prevent and cure many cancers.

Dr Oleg Chestnov, WHO Assistant Director-General for
Noncommunicable Diseases and Mental Health, Russia

Mum's story

My mother is a classic example of how lifestyle changes can make a priceless difference to someone's life.

In 2005, Mum suffered a heart attack. I rushed to Christchurch to spend time with her. Mum was basically told that she would be sick forever and to keep taking the drugs.

She was stressed, out of routine, overweight, and eating the wrong sorts of food. When she came out of hospital the specialists told her to 'take the drugs for the rest of your life as you are now at high risk of another heart attack.' Mum took the drugs for around 18 months, during which time she suffered devastatingly negative side effects that included memory loss, depression, mental confusion, anxiety, digestive issues and a severe loss of confidence.

After the 18 months had passed, she asked me if she could 'do the Jason stuff' to see if it would help her. I was thrilled and touched, of course. We set about changing her routines, diet, exercise and lifestyle habits. Our aim was to get her off the medications that were giving rise to many other problems. We changed her doctor, got her off all the heart drugs and transformed her health. How? We changed her diet and lifestyle. She was in better shape five years after the attack than she had been in years.

Once off the drugs, Mum found she had a clearer head, slept well every night, had more physical energy (she started planting trees!), wasn't depressed or numb, was thinking about her future, and was able to take long trips without heightened anxiety. She was able to have her grandchildren (two very active little boys) for a week on her own for the first time, and has since had them every six months for weeks on her own and loved it. Being in Cheviot with her is one of their favourite treats in the world – they have an amazing time together!

However, over time, bad habits crept back in; Mum went off the good foods and exercise regime and eventually suffered another heart episode. It certainly was an upsetting and terrifying time, and we are glad she has come out the other side of it. I was thrilled to discover that the senior cardiac rehab nurse who cared for Mum in hospital had done thelifeplan® and now recommends it to her patients as a very effective and heart-friendly diet. Thankfully, Mum is now willingly under the advice of her son again and will be for the rest of her life!

Remember that your body is your own, and it's your right to choose your doctor. There are wonderful and smart doctors everywhere. Find one. Choose wisely. Doctors are amazing people with high expertise in life-saving drug therapy, but they are not all experts in diet, lifestyle or longevity. There was nothing but doom and gloom ahead for my mother had she continued to follow her doctor's advice. Instead, she was motivated to make changes and is now a completely different woman – physically, emotionally, mentally, spiritually and, as a grandmother. The kids just LOVE her.

> The current approach to heart disease focuses only on short-term risks ... What determines your heart disease risk at age 70 is your risk factors at age 40.
>
> Dr Jarett Berry, University of Texas Southwestern Medical Centre, USA

Cancer, heart disease and Western medicine

The top three causes of death in most Western countries are cancer, heart disease and Western medicine. For example, in the US the biggest cause of death is heart disease, at more than 700,000 each year. The second biggest cause of death is cancer, at more than 500,000 people. The third biggest cause of death is medical care[17] (mistakes by doctors[18] and adverse reactions[19] from **correctly** prescribed drugs or surgery), at 225,000[20] people. These are people dying from legal medicines or treatments that are supposed to be saving their lives.[21]

There are 99,000 deaths from hospital infections every year in the US alone. These are infections caught **after** going to hospital. On any given day, some 80,000 patients in Europe are fighting an infection they caught in hospital, meaning hospital infections affect 3.2 million people in Europe every year.[22]

Drug testing and effectiveness exposed

During a decade as Head of Global Cancer Research at Amgen, C. Glenn Begley identified 53 important publications and papers in top journals. He sought to double-check the findings before trying to build on them for drug development. Despite his best people working on them, 47 of the 53 could not be replicated. 'It was shocking. These are the studies the pharmaceutical industry relies on to identify new targets for drug development.'[23] In a 2011 paper titled, 'Believe it or Not', scientists at Bayer analysed 'exciting published data' from basic science studies. Bayer scientists worked full time for up to a year trying to reproduce findings in 47 cancer research projects. Less than a quarter of the findings were able to be replicated.

4

How do we get from where we are, to where we want to be?

> You either change and pay a small proactive amount for your health now or you will pay a dramatically larger amount for your sickness and healthcare later on. If you want to improve your life then improve your diet. An improved diet changes the bacteria in your gut, changes your genetic expression towards health, and rebuilds your brain proteins. This changes your emotions and willpower and improves your decisions, thus improving your life and dramatically lowering your risk of depression, heart disease, obesity, diabetes and lifestyle cancers.
>
> Jason Shon Bennett

People are threatened by change

Not too long ago, people were 100% clear that the world was flat. Imagine the first person who stood up and dared to say: 'I think the world isn't flat, it's round, we are not the centre of the universe, we are just one of a bunch of planets circling this big gaseous fireball.' Can you imagine if the Internet was available then – what dialogue would have occurred? What thunderous objection would have rained down on that person? Overnight, thousands of websites have been created to give conclusive evidence that the author was wrong: the world is flat, we can prove it is flat (just watch this video!), and the author has just misrepresented the facts and twisted the study to suit his theory, and is a fruit-loop nut-job.

> Use three physicians still: first, Doctor Quiet,
> next Doctor Merryman, and finally, Doctor Diet.
>
> Constantin the African

A paradigm shift

Well, the world is round. Knowing this has enabled us to understand gravity, space and science much more effectively. We learnt about the seasons and how the moon impacts on ocean tides, and why we have daylight and night time. Once people fully understood the galaxy, their understanding of the world literally changed overnight. This is called a paradigm shift.

It is exactly the same with your body. Once you understand what food does to the body and how much better you can feel every day, it is far easier to make the change. Fortunately, we do not have to agree blindly that the world is flat anymore. Unfortunately, for many in the medical profession, the past is always present, which can be interpreted as meaning there's no room for change.

Fear rules before change happens

Throughout history outspoken proponents of new ideas who have dared to announce 'We could do this better' or 'I have discovered something that goes against what we all thought and believed' have been ridiculed. They were often thrown out of prestigious institutions, run out of town and subjected to media smear campaigns.

Israeli scientist Daniel Shechtman is one of those people. He discovered quasicrystals (patterns in atoms which were thought impossible). When he announced his discovery in 1982, his colleagues mocked him, insulted him, and exiled him from his research group. After years in the scientific wilderness, his assertions were proven correct. As a result, Shectman's discovery has changed the way the world sees the very nature of the matter all around us. In October 2011, he received the ultimate personal and public vindication: the Nobel Prize for Chemistry, for this discovery. His colleagues were, quite simply, afraid of change.

> For the two out of three adult Americans who do not smoke and
> do not drink excessively, one personal choice seems to influence
> long-term health prospects more than any other: what we eat.
>
> The US Surgeon-General's Report on Nutrition and Health, 1988

Change is always challenged

A German philosopher named Arthur Schopenhauer (1788–1860) made an incredibly insightful statement about human nature (and ironically, big business). He said, 'All truth goes through three stages. First, it is ridiculed. Second, it is violently opposed. Finally, it is accepted as self evident.'

This formula can be applied to cigarette smoking. In 1932, two studies proved smoking was one cause of lung cancer. However, evidence that claimed smoking made people sick was ridiculed and the messengers were sued or blacklisted. In 1992, 60 years later, the truth about smoking, that it kills 50% of all smokers (and hundreds of thousands of innocent bystanders every year, including children), was accepted. Smoking is now recognised as having been the biggest cause of preventable death in the last 100 years, killing over 100 million people needlessly. Remember, tobacco companies had evidence that cigarettes were harmless …

If you read a study telling you that soft drinks or junk foods are healthy, remember that the world is flat, and that has been proven too! Just as the tobacco studies showed 'cigarettes have no relationship to lung cancer', any studies that question the role junk foods play in our health problems will be heavily biased and funded by the global junk food industry.

I am resigned to the fact that much of what I have to say will be ridiculed because it goes against the current orthodox medical thinking that drugs will save you; you need to eat lots of meat to be healthy; or your diet has no influence on illness. In fact, I recommend the complete opposite.

Remember, when there's no way a message can be undermined, the messenger will bear the brunt of the attack. Victor Crawford, a tobacco lobbyist turned tobacco control advocate admitted that he, 'coined the phrase, "Health Nazis". I used the oldest trick in the book. When there's no way you can attack the message, attack the messenger. There was no way I could attack anything advocates said about health and addiction and win. It wasn't even an option. So I'd always say, "Well, the jury's still out on the health stuff, but that's not the real issue. The real issue is freedom of choice, and these health Nazis want to take it away!"'

Victor died of lung cancer, regretting his comments. He was only 63.

> Why is it that anything on this earth we do not understand,
> we are pushed down on our knees, to worship or to damn?
>
> Matt Johnson, 'The Violence of Truth' from the album
> *Mind Bomb* by The The, UK, 1989

Being attacked for telling the truth

I foresee being run down on talkback radio shows and during television discussions by scientific 'experts' paid by the food industry to promote the addictive mix of sugar, salt, fat and gluten. Sadly, I predict I may even be criticised by cancer and heart disease foundations for suggesting that food is the crucial element in disease prevention. However, I recall important facts, such as one from Frederick L. Hoffman, who founded the American Cancer Society (ACS) in 1913. Hoffman made it clear that he believed that 'diet was the way to prevent and treat cancer.' Diet, not drugs.

The modern diet is toxic

In the words of the great economist Lord John Maynard Keynes, 'When the facts change, I change my mind. What do you do, sir?'

Well, the facts have changed and the extent to which the typical modern diet does not work is clear for everyone to see. Obesity, diabetes, cancers, heart disease, asthma, osteoporosis, mental disorders, depression, serious digestive conditions and arthritis are all rife. Bizarrely, you can sit in your doctor's office, when you are sick (again), and read magazines and even medical journals that are littered with adverts for Coca Cola, McDonald's, KFC, fast foods, junk foods, takeaways, lollies and fried, rancid foods of the worst kind. Nobody thinks anything of it, yet this is exactly what is causing the problem. If you are admitted to hospital, it's standard practice to be asked if you drink alcohol or smoke. However, you are not asked about the single biggest influence on your health: your diet.[1]

New Zealand is built on a farm

I may be attacked by dietitians working for the food industry. After all, in terms of the economy, New Zealand is one big farm. We depend on meat and dairy sales to fuel our income. Senior researchers and concerned food scientists may say my research is flawed, that I am an extremist nutcase. They may insist my findings are idiotic, extreme and unsustainable. I may be vilified and dismissed as a nobody fruit-loop quack.

However, the doctor whose opinion I care for the most is a very old and very wise old geezer by the name of Hippocrates. He said, 'Let food be thy medicine.' These words have stood the test of time and they are more true and more needed now than they ever have been at any time in history.

> Diseases are likely to build up over a much longer period
> of time than was previously thought. It has changed the
> way we think about how ageing-related diseases develop.
>
> Researchers and chemists at the Australian National University, 2011

The story of Jack LaLanne

For many years doctors ridiculed Francois Henri 'Jack' LaLanne, a US longevity and fitness expert. They claimed that his ideas had no scientific basis. Those doctors are now all dead. Jack lived a long and healthy life, was in great shape and did crazy things like exercising right up to his death at nearly 100. Jack once described himself at various times as being 'a miserable goddamn junk food junkie sugarholic kid with a bad temper, headaches and bulimia.' When he was 15, Paul Bragg kicked off his nutritional education by explaining to him 'the evils of meat and sugar.'

LaLanne set about changing his life. He started eating very good quality food and exercising. At 54, he whipped 21-year-old Arnold Schwarzenegger in an informal contest of strength. He opened the first ever 'health gym' in 1936 in California, even though local doctors 'advised ... patients to stay away from his health club and warned ... that LaLanne was an exercise nut whose programs would cause severe medical problems such as heart attacks and loss of their sex drive ...'

A long healthy life based on good food and eating less

Walter Breuning died peacefully in February 2011 aged 114 years. At the time, he was the world's oldest man. He stopped eating dinner in 1979. His doctors warned him against it and told him he would die soon. He lived for another 30 years in stunning health. His doctors died young.

The world's oldest man ever is Jiroemon Kimura, who turned 116 on 19 April 2013. He is officially the oldest recorded man in history. He said his secret to longevity was a strict plant-based diet of rice, vegetables, miso soup, porridge, red beans and fish. He never smoked and rarely drank alcohol. His secret was 'to eat three small meals per day, and to stop eating when his stomach is about 80% full.' He walked most days and he still had normal blood pressure at 116 (remember, the number one cause of death in the world is high blood pressure, a condition suffered by many 40-year-olds).

My Granny Amy lived to 104. She weathered criticisms and storms about her strict vegetarian diet and lifestyle, but she endured. She died peacefully in her sleep of old age, the way we all dream of dying.

When it comes to preventing disease and increasing drug-free longevity, modern medicine has nothing to match lifestyle changes. Only changing your lifestyle will cure a lifestyle disease. **You cannot eat yourself sick and then drug yourself well.**

Even experts are human and need help

I have helped nurses with their diverticulitis, doctors with their diets, naturopaths with their allergies, dietitians with weight loss, social workers with their stress levels, and pharmacists and chemists with their blood pressure, fertility, skin, bowel and sleeping problems. All of my help has been in the form of dietary and lifestyle changes. I do not pretend to be a doctor. I offer something different: prevention. Even if you are well, you can always improve your health, your lifestyle and your habits.

The simple things are the most powerful

My recommendations for health and longevity are:

- ▶ a healthy, fresh, plant-based wholefood diet that includes lots of local vegetation, fruits, vegetables, nuts and seeds and correctly prepared legumes and wholegrains (with some occasional fresh fish or good quality eggs if desired)
- ▶ eating less overall
- ▶ regular fasting
- ▶ daily movement, especially walking
- ▶ get more sleep, particularly before 10 pm
- ▶ rest
- ▶ relaxation, for example breathing exercises and/or meditation
- ▶ more water, less or no coffee.
- ▶ low or zero alcohol intake (NB, two glasses of wine every night is not 'low'!).

I recommend you see vegetable carbohydrates as the single most important component of your diet. Meat, dairy, alcohol and processed foods are special treats (if at all). These positive changes to your diet, lifestyle and environment will change your energy levels, your weight problems, your skin, your vitality, your sex drive, your health profile, your disease risk and your longevity.

You are in charge of your health

You will see why I recommend these things as this book progresses. You can take the power away from the big food and drug companies and return it to yourself, where it belongs. The food and drug industries will not like my message, as they make trillions of dollars per year peddling their wares. They will fight the PR war to continue to feed you their junk foods, sugar drinks, cigarettes and alcohol to keep you sick, overweight and brain dead, and then they will sell you drugs for your lifestyle disease, which the drugs will not cure. This cycle makes them a staggering amount of money.

It is good for them. But it is not good for you.

Step back from the advertising hype

Once you look at something objectively from different angles, and you ask the hard questions and try to prove a theory wrong; once you remove your emotional attachment to the result; and once you remove the big business marketing and advertising we are all subjected to, you can see things more clearly. Once you remove the need to sell something, then you have the basis for accurate and proven advice that works.

This book is based on nearly 30 years of research, eight long years of writing and access to tens of thousands of hours of studies about millions of people in countries across the world. Once I had cured my own illness and seen my suggestions work on many others, it became crystal clear to me that modern medicine offers great pills and procedures after you get sick. But I have the benefit of a long-term view.

I can offer prevention. I base my advice on the best science, research and long-term epidemiological studies I can find.

The considerable research

My research references include the following. More references are listed at jasonshonbennett.com.

▶ An Evaluation of Research in the United States on Human Nutrition, Report No. 2: Benefits from Nutrition Research

▶ Framingham Heart Study, 1960–ongoing

- The 351-page 2012 World Cancer Report
- The Annual Global Burden of Disease Studies, 2008–2010
- The Cancer Atlas Survey
- The European Prospective Investigation into Cancer and Nutrition (EPIC) Study
- The Harvard Nurses' Health Study I & II, 1984–2013
- The Initiation of the US Dietary Guidelines, 1980
- The Malmo Diet and Cancer Study
- The Multiple Risk Factor Intervention Trial (MRFIT)
- The National Academy of Sciences (NAS) report on Diet, Nutrition and Cancer, 1982
- The National Health and Nutrition Examination Survey (NHANES)
- The National Institutes of Health-AARP Diet and Health Study
- World Cancer Research Fund

Peer reviewed studies

In my research I have read hundreds of papers, studies and clinical research ranging from the 1800s to the present day. These come from reputable journals and other scientific publications and include the following titles.

Archives of Internal Medicine

Archives of Neurology

BMC Genomics

British Medical Journal

Carcinogenesis and Cancer

CardioSmart (College of Cardiology)

Circulation (US Heart Association)

Clinical Cancer Research

Hepatology

Journal of Chronic Disease

Journal of Clinical Endocrinology

Journal of Nutrition

Lancet Oncology

Life Sciences

Metabolism

Nature

Nutrition and Cancer

PLOS ONE (Public Library of Science)

The American Journal of Cardiology

The American Journal of Clinical Nutrition

The American Journal of Epidemiology

The International Journal of Cancer

The Journal of Family Practice

The Journal of the American Diet Association

The New England Journal of Medicine

The Scientist

Credible and published proof

The scientific studies I cite have been used and confirmed by, among others, the National Cancer Institute, The Centers for Disease Control and Prevention, The World Health Organization, National Academy of Sciences (NAS), American Institute for Cancer Research (AICR), The World Preservation Foundation (WPF), The International Union Against Cancer, as well as a long list of world-leading and highly credible practitioners and authors. These include ex-heart surgeon Dr Caldwell Esselstyn, Director of the Cardiovascular Prevention and Reversal Program in Cleveland Clinic Wellness Institute; Dr Dean Ornish, founder of the Preventive Medicine Research Institute (chosen by *Life* magazine as, 'one of the 50 most influential members of his generation'); Dr Neal Barnard, founder of the Physicians Committee for Responsible Medicine; Dr Joel Fuhrman, Director of Research for the Nutritional Research Project for the National Health Association; and the great T. Colin Campbell, author, the Jacob Gould Schurman Professor Emeritus of Nutritional Biochemistry at Cornell University, and lead scientist in the 1980s China-Oxford-Cornell study on diet and disease, set up in 1983 by Cornell University, the University of Oxford and the Chinese Academy of Preventive Medicine.

To know what you prefer instead of humbly saying Amen
to what the world tells you you ought to prefer,
is to have kept your soul alive.

Robert Louis Stevenson, author

Go Gary!

Robert Louis Stevenson's quote reminds me of a dear old friend of mine, Gary. Sadly, Gary passed away in July 2009. He was a champion for supporting people to change the world and follow their dreams. Gary would be the first to say, 'Just because something has been done the same way for a long time, it does not make it good, smart or effective.'

Well, here it is Gary; my dream, my first book (after being asked to write one for over 20 years). I always loved and admired your maverick attitude to life, and I bring that to this book!

Change is required

In life, change is often required, even if we do not want it! During my nearly 30 years of varied and exhaustive nutritional research and study, I have found strong scientific truths that have been proven to work countless times by millions of people all over the globe.

To gain these benefits you may have to change your habits, change the way you see the world and change the way you understand yourself. You may have to change your kitchen cupboards, change the time you go to bed, change the time you wake up, change what you do when you wake up, and change the way you see food.

I have discovered an effective method that will reverse illness, strengthen your body, reignite your energy, and help slow the aging process. Read this book, try it on: if you discover something works then keep doing it. If you try something and it doesn't work, throw it out and try the next suggestion.

In support of my theories, I use examples of what I have discovered, the research behind it, and the experience of traditional peoples (and how they stay healthy), and I try to bust a few myths along the way.

I give simple tips and easy summaries of small, everyday things you can do to improve your energy, health, longevity and skin and lower your risk of almost all modern non-communicable disease (NCDs). These include cancers, heart disease, autoimmune diseases, obesity and diabetes.

The fact that an opinion has been widely held is no evidence
whatever that it is not utterly absurd; indeed in view of the
silliness of the majority of mankind, a widespread belief
is more likely to be foolish than sensible.

Bertrand Russell, philospher

Health myths

Some of the things I suggest may be very unusual or strange concepts to you. Believe me, most of them sounded pretty whacky to me when I first encountered them. However, I now understand that doing something over and over again when it doesn't serve you is what is actually crazy. Changing your bad habits can create miracles. As Charles Darwin wisely said, 'It is not the strongest who survive, nor the most intelligent, but the ones most responsive to change.'

There are many so-called truths in the health industry that are really only about selling a product or a drug. I do not have products to sell you. My ambition is to share what I have learned, tell the story of what I have done, and make a genuine and profound difference to your health. My hope is that there are new solutions in this book for people who are not satisfied with where their health is currently at.

On a personal note, I do not suggest anything unless I believe in it 100%.

Happy, happy, joy, joy

My best ever friend, Rob, once asked me, 'What is the critical factor to long-term health?' I replied, 'Food, food, food, food, food, food, food and food. And exercise is good too.' He laughed and laughed and told me to put it in my book.

The thing is, I wasn't kidding! Exercise is a critical factor to your long-term health but what you are putting in your mouth is the cornerstone that **everything** else is built on, your fitness included. You do not eat exercise and build your body on exercise; you build your body, including your bones, skin, organs, immune system and bowels, on food.

Is my way the only way to get well?

Of course not! There are a lot of ways to eat well and get well. There are so many good foods and so many different cultures and philosophies that work wonders. My theory is what has worked for me when nothing else did. It has also helped thousands of people with whom I have worked.

Life should be a journey to the grave skidding in sideways,
a delicious drink in one hand, fresh strawberries in the other,
body completely used up, totally worn out and screaming,
'I did it all, woohoo, what a ride!'

Hunter S. Thompson (with a little artistic licence taken)

One last thing: get your attitude on!

Being healthy does not mean being a boring, righteous, sad-sack misery guts. I have a great life. I can dance and party longer than anyone I know (except maybe my old fitness buddy, Steve McGough). I laugh at everything. Life is way too short to be overly significant about food.

The truth is that great health is what we all really want. The energy and youthfulness of children is what we envy. Being healthy and vital means you have more energy to burn and a better ability to do the things you want to achieve in your life. I can prove that your diet and lifestyle have more power and influence over your health than anything modern medicine has to offer. I am advocating prevention.

This book is for people who are sick and tired of being sick and tired, and are willing to do something about it. I am a permanent health student and this book, for me, is a reminder that 'you teach best that which you most need to learn.'

5

Eat Less, Live Long

Man lives on a quarter of what he eats.
On the other three-quarters his doctor lives.

Carved into a 3800-year-old Egyptian pyramid

You can have a healthy, long life

Do you want to live into your 80s, 90s or 100s with great health and vitality, without disease? Yes, of course! We all do, but most of us are deeply cynical. We have seen our grandparents suffer into their 80s and we believe it is a normal part of the aging process to get sick as we get older. We have a programmed belief that the last 30 years of our lives are automatically going to consist of illness and poor health. We imagine that the power to do anything about it is totally out of our hands. The truth is somewhat different. Science proves that almost 200 things can slow aging in humans. Of those, you can change 150 of these aspects of your health through the power you have over your own genetic expression.

The way to eat a lot is to eat little, that way you
live long enough to be able to eat a lot.

Anonymous

Live to 100 in great shape?

Would living to 100 without illness, with a sharp mind, and being able to take care of yourself, be appealing to you? Of course! Would you like the absolute privilege of getting to know your sixteenth great-grandchild and watching them grow and create a family of their own? Of course you would! The simple things in life bring the greatest pleasure.

Today there are around half a million centenarians in the world. The message? Be 'wellderly', not elderly. If you would like to improve your chances of a long and healthy life dramatically, then eating less, or rather, eating the right amount for the human body, is the most powerful and scientifically proven way to extend your lifespan.

People eating one-third less than the typical Western diet live up to 50% longer, and in much better health. The typical modern diet is around 3000 calories of nutrient poor, low fibre, sugar-rich refined carbohydrates, highly processed animal foods and toxic rancid fats. On average, all we actually require daily is around 1800 calories of high fibre, nutrient rich, plant-based wholefoods.

Overeating causes oxidative damage, which causes your DNA to age. Eating less food and eating better quality food results in less DNA damage. High fibre foods that are rich in 'plantioxidants' (my name for the powerful protector-nutrient antioxidants found only in plant foods), such as vegetables, fruits, nuts and seeds, all reduce oxidation and maximise our natural enzyme protection systems. Limiting DNA damage is vital if we are trying to improve our quality of life, live longer, and prevent major chronic lifestyle illnesses such as osteoporosis, arthritis, diabetes, obesity, heart disease, asthma, mental decline and cancer.

Why make a big deal about staying in shape?

The truth is that the causality between being overweight and diabetes is the same as the causality between smoking and lung cancer. If current worldwide trends continue, one in three of all children born after the year 2000 will suffer from type II diabetes.

All people who live long, regardless of nationality, race or gender, share one thing in common: none are overweight.

Dr Shigeaki Hinohara, age 97,
one of the world's longest-serving doctors

Overeating and eating the wrong sorts of foods that do not serve the human body is the most effective way to raise your risk of almost all disease; unfortunately this behaviour is a trained, advertised and marketed habit of our environment. Being overweight with diabetes is now the prime cause of illness, leading to 34 different cancers, hypertension, heart disease, heart attacks, limb amputations, blindness, gall stones and strokes.

The Golden Rule is to Eat Less

Eating a third less than average while maintaining a full and complete nutritional intake will give you:

▶ more energy, vitality and stamina

▶ reduced lifestyle-fat content (this is the deadliest kind)

▶ sustained long-term weight loss giving a healthier and leaner weight

▶ a more powerful and effective immune system

▶ a happier digestive system with more stable blood-glucose levels

▶ a sharper mind with a much lower risk of brain diseases

▶ instant improvement in your DNA health

▶ lower body-acidity levels

▶ decreased inflammation, protecting you from almost all illness

▶ an immediate slowing of the aging process.

Eating less: my experience

One of the first things I did when I embarked on my journey to cure myself was a seven-day fast. What became apparent very quickly was how little sleep I needed, how clear my skin became, and how much more energy I had. I got an absolute glow on. My body was finally being given a holiday from all the overeating.

This led me to ask myself, 'What would happen if I just cut back the amount of food I ate every day?' Let me be very clear here, I am **not** talking about starving myself. I am talking about eating the right amount of nutrition my body required to function at optimal levels. I discovered I was eating too much and this was stressing my entire system. Once you start to feel the benefits of eating less, you then wonder why we eat so much and you realise that we mainly eat for our emotional state, not the health or longevity of our body. Throughout history we have eaten around 1800 to 2000 calories per day. And that was only when fresh food was available!

Overeating kills you slowly

Both laboratory rats and humans will eat to obesity when there is enough food around them. When you overeat it makes you tired and sluggish (both mentally and physically), increases acidity, stresses the body, accelerates aging, makes you fat and sets off a chain reaction that weakens all your internal organs. Today's centenarians (people who live to be 100 years old) would never have eaten to excess. When you are overweight, you are actually malnourished at the same time that you are overfed.

> We are recommending that people aim to be as lean as possible (within the healthy range) and that they avoid weight gain throughout adulthood. The fact is that putting on weight can increase your cancer risk. This report's recommendations represent the most definitive advice on preventing cancer that has ever been available anywhere in the world.
>
> World Cancer Research Fund, 2007

A healthy life expectancy is declining rapidly, not growing

Overeating, poor diet and sedentary lifestyles are the indisputable contributing factors to high death rates from heart disease. Even though our life expectancy is currently increasing slightly, our last 30 years are generally full of illness and suffering. As we have already seen, the myth that we are living longer and healthier lives is untrue. It has been proven incorrect by economic institutions, scientists, doctors and epidemiologists. We are getting sicker at a younger age with every generation. The average age at which heart disease strikes is getting lower every year, just as its incidence is increasing every year. The same is happening all over the world with liver cancer, breast cancer, prostate cancer, lung cancer, osteoporosis, asthma, obesity and diabetes.

Born after 2000? Expect to be a diabetic!

Tragically, our own kids, the current generation of obese children, are not expected to live as long as we do. In 2008, Diabetes UK boldly claimed that life expectancy in Britain will start falling for the first time in 200 years because of the rise in obesity and diabetes. Simply put, childhood obesity is leading to shorter lifespans. A study published in the *New England Journal of Medicine* in February 2010 suggested children today will live an average two to five years less than their parents and grandparents. This is a preventable, early, painful-death effect equal to all cancer deaths combined.

We hear all the time about how we are living longer lives, but the truth is that we are living sicker lives longer. According to the International Longevity Centre UK (ILC-UK), less than one in three of us will reach age 65 in good health.[1] That means 30% of us will be healthy at age 65, and 70% of us will be sick. If you want to know how long you are predicted to live in good health, you can believe Paul McCartney: it's 64.

The potential human lifespan remains at 120 years (which some people can approach in good health), but the sad truth is that we are dying in our 60s and 70s after decades of preventable health problems.

Calorie restriction, but not nutrient restriction, leads to lower inflammatory biomarkers such as C reactive protein, IL6, fasting blood sugar, fasting insulin, LDL cholesterol and triglycerides. It also decreases visceral fat and reduces oxidative stress and damage. In non-human primates it decreases mortality due to type II diabetes, cardiovascular disease and cancer. Calorie restriction and exercise activates a metabolic pathway called 'Master Metabolic Regulator Pathway'. This ultimately leads to the production of new mitochondria, which means more effective, more efficient and sustained energy production with less oxidative stress.

Dr Ingrid Pincott, Naturopathic Doctor, Canada

Four elephants in a Mini

Imagine two Mini cars fresh from the manufacturing plant. They are genetic twins. Mini No. 1 is given the right amount of good fuel and is driven by one 70 kg human. It gets an oil change as required, is cleaned once a week and is not driven on Sundays, when it sits and relaxes in the garage, consuming no fuel and resting quietly.

Mini No. 2 is given low-quality fuel that does not serve the engine very well. It never gets an oil change. It is driven every day without a break and it has four elephants in it at all times. Each elephant weighs four tonnes. Imagine trying to drive this Mini with the four elephants. How far do you think you will get? How will the car handle? What is the car's life expectancy? How long before basic systems start to break down and stop working? How much extra money are you going to have to spend at the garage to keep it roadworthy?

Ask any good mechanic if Mini No. 1 will have a significantly longer life and be in really good shape and, of course, the answer would be 'yes'. It will last two to three times as long as the poor, overburdened Mini with the four elephants squashed into it. The mechanic will tell you Mini No. 2 will lose half its lifespan. It will spend most of its life in very poor shape, coughing and spluttering as it tries to haul the elephants around – much like a human being who constantly overeats.

Think of your body in exactly the same way. Are you Mini No. 1 or Mini No. 2? The choice is yours.

> None of us, probably, want another five years in a nursing
> home, but an additional five years without any particular
> health problems would be another matter.

Linda Partridge, Director of University College London's Institute of Healthy Aging

Eat yourself to longevity or to the hospital

When we eat less on a plant-based wholefood diet our DNA changes. This calorie restriction (CR) is defined as 'a reduction in energy intake without malnutrition'. The aging process slows, the body has maximum energy, the immune system functions better, and our digestive tracts expel waste two or three times daily. Eating less, but nutrient-rich food, leads to longevity, youthful energy levels, super-health, a very low risk of disease and a vastly improved quality of life.

When you constantly overeat your engine becomes worn out in half the time of someone who does not constantly overeat. You lose your youthful mobility, your systems break down and you are more often than not at the doctor's spending money on drugs that will not fix the problem. When we consistently overeat we build up acidity, so we need more and more plantioxidants to clear the acidity from the body. We develop an overburdened digestive system, which leads to lower nutritional absorption, bowel problems and constipation. This leads to a stressed and struggling liver and a weakened immune system. We start to run on less energy, and we become more toxic, more constipated and sick. Our skin (the biggest eliminative organ we have) starts to age prematurely, and lose its glow, and our body starts slowly to break down and fall apart. All these problems arise from long-term consistent overeating.

Eating less is actually eating normally

The best way to slow aging is to eat less. This is not starvation or some type of eating disorder. I am not talking about a low calorie diet, but rather a 'normal for human beings throughout history' calorie diet. This will vary from person to person, as we all eat slightly differently, and that is fine. The key is to eat for your body, not your emotions. The right calorie intake for your body requirements is what you need to discover. You may find your required amount is far less than you ever thought it could be. Wrong calories belong to the modern, high calorie, low fibre, low nutrition diets we now all live on.

Eating less protects life

Eating less induces beneficial metabolic, hormonal and functional changes for maximum longevity.[2] It enhances your longevity, partly by reducing visceral abdominal fat. Visceral abdominal fat is responsible for inflammation and leads to chronic disease. Eating less improves physiological function and performance and slows the progression of physical disability in age. This has significant longevity-enhancing implications for humans.[3] What has been identified and shown, is how this process of 'eating less' actually works to increase lifespan dramatically.[4]

Eating less, or calorie restriction, changes the genetic activity of the nutrient-sensing pathway, inducing a mechanism that slows aging.

6
Calorie restriction

Obesity prevents longevity.

Dr Leonid Gavrilov, National Insitute of Health researcher,
University of Chicago

Cell telomeres and longevity

Telomeres protect the end of your chromosomes from deterioration. The
name 'telomere' comes from the words 'end' and 'root', as in the end of the
beginning of life. Without telomeres our genomes would forget who and
what they are and their function. As each telomere cell divides, the telomere
ends become shorter and less healthy. The shorter your telomeres and the
faster they break down, the higher your risk of high blood pressure and early
death.

Eating less slows the breakdown of your cell chromosome telomeres.
People with a simply modified growth hormone receptor seldom suffer
from diabetes or tumours. Mice on a restricted calorie intake have a reduced
number of senescent cells in both the liver and the intestines (where they
accumulate with aging), lower cancer rates, and better preserved telomeres
than mice that eat more liberally.[1] The restricted food intake protects the
telomeres. We have also seen this in many studies in humans. In a study
of over 3500 people with heart disease, monitoring revealed that telomere
length predicted their survival rates better than any other measure.[2] Almost
2000 people were studied and their telomere length was linked with the early

onset of dementia.[3] In 1600 people studied, shorter telomeres correlated with higher rates of depression.[4]

> For most of human evolution we have lived on a local plant-based fresh, raw, soaked, sprouted, fermented and cooked wholefood diet. We have survived regular periods of scarcity with fasting because there was not a fridge in every house or cave, or a McDonald's on every street corner.
>
> Jason Shon Bennett

Eating less in the animal kingdom

The first clinical experiments in eating less were performed on rats by Clive M. McCay and Mary F. Crowell in November 1934 at Cornell University, New York. They discovered that every creature, regardless of age, when fed a restricted but nutritionally complete food intake, lived almost twice as long as those with unrestricted access to food. Not only that, the animals were stronger and far more resistant to all of the usual diseases. Follow-up studies on yeast cells, worms, mice, spiders, bacteria, guinea pigs, dogs and then monkeys revealed the same results as those obtained by McCay and Crowell.

Worms to primates

Worms on a cycle of fasting and feeding outlast their relatives by 19 generations while maintaining youthful physiological traits. All animals fed a lower calorie diet lived longer, partly because their cells could resist stress better, the researchers said. Eating less primes the body to resist the more severe stresses that cause cells to age. Scientists have long known that, in animals studied, a 40–60% reduction in calorie intake, while maintaining a healthy diet of nutrient rich foods, consistently prolongs life by up to 40%. This regime also reduces the risk of cancer, diabetes and heart disease, while staving off age-related degeneration of the brain and nervous system. All scientists agreed there were huge potential payoffs in reducing calorie intake while maintaining a healthy diet rich in plant-based phytonutrients.[5]

The 1989–2012 Wisconsin National Primate Research Center Calorie Restriction Study

At the University of Wisconsin at Madison, 75 adult Rhesus monkeys were divided into two groups. One group ate a normal, unrestricted healthy diet. The second group ate the same diet, but were given 30% less food. The calorie-restricted monkeys showed no evidence of diabetes, which usually affects about 50% of normal monkeys in captivity; they had reduced brain atrophy; and their risk of developing cardiovascular disease and cancer was significantly lower. They also had much less body fat than their unrestricted counterparts, so they were potentially protected against a wide range of illnesses including heart disease, cancer and obesity.

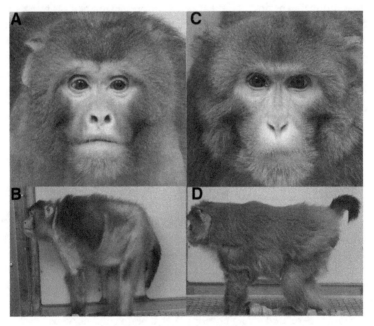

Both monkeys are aged 27. They ate the same healthy, balanced diet, but the one on the right ate 30% less. The differences are staggering. Photo: Jeff Miller.

From Colman, Ricki J., Anderson, Rozalyn M., Johnson, Sterling C., Kastman, Erik K., Kosmatka, Kristopher J., Beasley, T. Mark, Allison, David B., Cruzen, Christina, Simmons, Heather A., Kemnitz, Joseph, W., and Weindruch, Richard, 'Caloric Restriction Delays Disease Onset and Mortality in Rhesus Monkeys', in *Science*, The American Association for the Advancement of Science, Issue 5937, Volume 325, 10 July 2009. Reprinted with permission from AAAS.

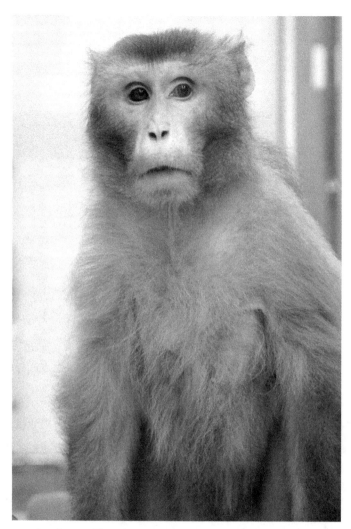

Rhesus monkey Canto, 27, and on a restricted diet, is pictured at the Wisconsin National Primate Research Center at the University of Wisconsin-Madison on 28 May 2009. Photo: Jeff Miller.

From Colman, Ricki J., Anderson, Rozalyn M., Johnson, Sterling C., Kastman, Erik K., Kosmatka, Kristopher J., Beasley, T. Mark, Allison, David B., Cruzen, Christina, Simmons, Heather A., Kemnitz, Joseph, W., and Weindruch, Richard, 'Caloric Restriction Delays Disease Onset and Mortality in Rhesus Monkeys', in *Science*, The American Association for the Advancement of Science, Issue 5937, Volume 325, 10 July 2009. Reprinted with permission from AAAS.

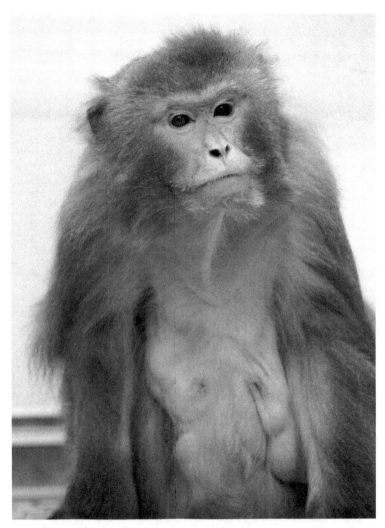

Rhesus monkey Owen, 29, and a control subject on an unrestricted diet, is pictured at the Wisconsin National Primate Research Center at the University of Wisconsin-Madison on 28 May 2009. Photo: Jeff Miller.

From Colman, Ricki J., Anderson, Rozalyn M., Johnson, Sterling C., Kastman, Erik K., Kosmatka, Kristopher J., Beasley, T. Mark, Allison, David B., Cruzen, Christina, Simmons, Heather A., Kemnitz, Joseph, W., and Weindruch, Richard, 'Caloric Restriction Delays Disease Onset and Mortality in Rhesus Monkeys', in *Science*, The American Association for the Advancement of Science, Issue 5937, Volume 325, 10 July 2009. Reprinted with permission from AAAS.

Monkeys with unrestricted food	Monkeys eating 30% less (same food)
14 deaths from age-related disease	5 deaths from age-related disease
11 pre-diabetic conditions	0 pre-diabetic conditions
High cardiovascular and cancer rates	50% lower cardiovascular and cancer rates

The research revealed that, 'the calorie-restricted monkeys were less likely to get heart disease, diabetes, cancer or other diseases of aging. By 2009, 80% of the non-dieting Wisconsin monkeys had died of age-related illness; only 50% of dieting monkeys had.'[6]

The results were indisputable, clear and categorical. The monkeys that ate less lived much longer, in far better health, with very little disease or illness of any sort. Writing in *Science*, the US researchers hailed the major effect of the diet. Rhesus monkeys share 93% of our genes. If it works so well for them, surely we can learn to take heed and apply the science to the amount we eat?

> It's almost entirely obesity. How fat you are is the top and bottom of it. Not only is the overall incidence of diabetes increasing but the proportion of people aged 40 or less [with diabetes] rose markedly.
>
> Professor Craig Currie, School of Medicine, Cardiff University, Wales, June 2013

An additional and supporting study by the 2012 National Institute on Aging found that most of the 57 calorie-restricted monkeys had healthier hearts and immune systems, and lower rates of diabetes, cancer or other illnesses than the 64 monkeys eating as much as they liked. In 2012, in an analysis of the study for *Nature*, biologist Steven Austad of the University of Texas Health Science Center's Barshop Institute for Longevity and Aging Studies said, 'You can argue that the calorie-restricted animals are healthier, they have better cholesterol profiles, less muscle loss and less disease.'

Good for the monkey, good for the human?

The results of both the National Institute on Aging and Wisconsin studies show that monkeys eating less overall were healthier and stronger with less disease, and that age-related diseases occurred later in their lives. Because we share around 99% of our genes with chimpanzees, apes and orangutans, these studies point to a similar positive effect being possible in humans. All primates are designed to eat good quality, fresh, seasonally grown local foods, a diet high in plant vegetation and variety, and not too much. When presented with too many calories, primates, like humans will overeat. Not rocket science is it? Humans are good at dealing with famine. What we are not good at is dealing with too much food.

In June 2012, scientists from Washington University in St Louis published research showing that people on calorie-restricted diets had hearts that function, 'more like those found in people two decades younger.' Dr Luigi Fontana, who has studied calorie-restricted volunteers for eight years at the university, commented to the *Los Angeles Times* that 'mild caloric restriction is beneficial to everybody.' His experience has been that 'those who eat 30% less than average have the heart function of adults 16 years younger. The life extending genetic pathway is set off by dietary restriction.'

Sirtuins

Humans, primates, worms and mice retain many genetic mechanisms in common. One is the insulin-signalling control of metabolism and the ancient survival mechanism of riding out famines: the calorie restriction response. Basically, when you eat less, protein enzymes called sirtuins are activated by the body's response to having less energy. These sirtuins boost the rate of cell repair and cell regeneration, and dramatically slow the aging process. Sirtuins play a vital role in longevity and stress response. The sirtuin SIRT1 suppresses the production of amyloid beta proteins, which form plaques in the brains of Alzheimer's patients,[7] and blocks the development of prostate cancer.[8]

The longevity gene works – but you must eat correctly

The SIR2 gene is found in the human body. It can slow aging and stop age-related diseases such as diabetes, Alzheimer's, Parkinson's, heart disease and cancer. The great news is that it is not up to chance. The SIR2 gene is found in all human beings! However, the SIR2 gene is triggered only by a healthy, low calorie diet. Eating too much or eating the high calorie, typical modern diet adversely impacts the SIR2 gene, meaning it is not able to protect the body from diseases and rapid aging.[9]

> Our study resolves the role of SIR2 as a longevity gene.
> We have found that it may slow down the ageing process,

but a low calorie intake has a significant impact on SIR2 protein and helps the body combat age-related diseases.

Dr Ullas Kolthur, Tata Institute of Fundamental Research,
Department of Biological Sciences, Mumbai, India

Other genes

The enzymatic gene SIRT3 has a direct anti-aging effect, acting on the mitochondria. Mitochondria are structures inside the cells that produce energy, and reactive forms of oxygen called free radicals as a byproduct. Free radical DNA damage causes aging and sickness. When you eat less, SIRT3 levels increase, altering the metabolism of the body and slowing the aging process, showing that calorie resistance, aging and longevity tend to go hand in hand. This has been proven in humans.[10] However, sirtuins are not the golden longevity drug. They are part of myriad components – for example, eating less and eating a plant-based wholefood diet – that work together to protect and extend healthy lifespans.[11]

The live long and cure diabetes gene?

The Fox family of genes is a large family of master regulator genes that control other genes. They directly link eating fewer calories to living longer. The gene has exact counterparts in mammals. The three genes in mice and in people are known as FoxA 1, 2 and 3. These Fox genetic commanders work by regulating the food consumption between the extremes of harm caused by starvation and/or overeating.

Calorie restriction works for humans and lab rats as they both live under the same conditions: 75% of male rats and nearly 66% of female rats are overweight or obese, they have access to cheap, energy-dense food 24 hours a day, their offspring reach reproductive age younger due to overeating and they get very little exercise. Sounds like modern society to me.

Jason Shon Bennett

Not enough food

Longevity was significantly advanced when researchers 'switched on' or made more of the FoxA genes within worms. Not only did the worms live 50% longer, but the genes made them super-healthy and increased the removal of free radicals.[12] In less complex organisms, restricting calories doubles or triples lifespan. Just one FOXO gene, called DAF-16, has a massive impact on longer life expectancy, increases stress resistance and improves immunity against infections in worms.[14-25] Mice live 30% longer if fed a healthy low calorie diet.[13] Eating less has repeatedly been shown to cure type II diabetes within weeks, to the point where no more insulin is required, when combined with a high fibre, plant-based, wholefood diet.[14]

> It is striking to see how a relatively simple intervention of a very low calorie diet effectively cures type II diabetes mellitus. These effects are long-term, illustrating the potential of this method.
>
> Dr Sebastiaan Hammer, Department of Radiology,
> Leiden University Medical Center, Netherlands

To test the effect of calorie restriction on diabetics, Dutch researchers enlisted 15 obese men and women with type II diabetes. They were given a thorough physical check for fatty deposits in the heart (as they impair cardiac function). The volunteers followed a 500-calorie-a-day diet for four months. After four months their hearts were rescanned. Reasearchers found:

▶ the volume of pedicardial fat fell significantly, from 39 millilitres to 31 millilitres

▶ the 'E/A ratio', a common measure of cardiac function, rose from 0.96 to 1.2 (the lower the number, the higher the risk of heart failure)

▶ BMI fat fell from 35.3 to 27.5%

▶ the benefits of calorie restriction persisted after the volunteers went back to their usual eating habits and regained weight

▶ every volunteer was able to discontinue their insulin injections after embarking on calorie restriction.[15]

Eat less and trigger longevity

The Fox gene may be the primordial gene that regulates nutrients and helps us live a long time through dietary restriction. How do you trigger it? Eat less. As long as nutritional intake is adequate, then eating less causes reductions in almost all lifestyle disease factors, **even when restriction starts mid-life.** For humans, eating less causes the same metabolic adaptations that occur in animal studies. Other longevity genes lie in the insulin-signalling pathway, which influences your fat and glucose metabolism. This is also directly influenced by what and how much you eat. If you eat less, the insulin-signalling pathway activates a powerful gene regulator that controls many genetic pathways, and governs metabolism and your immune system.[16]

Eating less reduces oxidative damage from free radicals, slows aging, improves mitochondria function (the energy you have at a cellular level) and reduces DNA damage in skeletal tissue. This increases life expectancy and the quality of life by reducing the burden of chronic disease. You can add 25 years to your lifespan by eating less, eating better foods and exercising.[17] This is something worth considering right? Becoming wellderly, not elderly?

Does it work on humans?

Yes! Dr Maoshing Ni, a 38th generation doctor and author specialising in longevity, examined the diets of 100 centenarians and found that 'undereating was the norm.' The centenarians lived on a variety of legumes, whole grains, vegetables, fruits, nuts, seeds and very little meat. They walked at least 30 minutes daily; most walked more than an hour.

Eating less leads to a reduction in body weight, decreases the risk of type II diabetes, hypertension, cardiovascular disease, dementia, stroke, arthritis, gallstones, infertility, asthma, cataracts and cancers of the breast, prostate, kidney, liver and colon. Why would you not want to do it?

7
The longest-lived people in the world

Human studies

The first studies on the effects of caloric reduction on humans were done in the 1940s. The Scandinavian subjects of the study lived on a diet where their calories were restricted by 20% because of the hardships of the Second World War. They complained, but they also experienced a significant decrease in cardiovascular-related deaths. More research compared 18 members from the 'Calorie Restriction Society' to 18 healthy participants who ate a typical modern diet. The calorie restricted group scored far better in all major risk factors for heart disease and had 40% less plaque in their arteries.[1]

There are two great medicines: diet and self-control.

Oscar Maximilian Bircher-Benner, Swiss physician and nutritionist

The 1980s Biosphere Project

In the mid-1980s, an environmental experiment in the US was conducted where 25 volunteers lived in a hermetically sealed greenhouse for two years.[2]

Biosphere 2, a closed 1.2-hectare bubble in the Arizona desert, was designed to test whether the colonisation of space might be possible. They could not produce the amount of food they planned on, so everyone was rationed to 75% of their normal intake, which was a nutrient-rich diet of around 1800 calories daily. The results were astounding. Overall, they felt much better, their blood-pressure levels changed to match those of much younger people, and every single aging measure of blood, lipid, arteries and the immune system improved. Within six months their weights had fallen 14%, with dramatic improvements in blood pressure, cholesterol, blood sugar and insulin.

Lower blood pressure, lower body fat, sharper brain

The Washington School of Medicine study showed the average blood pressure of a group eating less was typical of 10-year-olds and their body fat was that of serious athletes. One of the group commented that 'headaches and colds are all gone; most of us seem to be able to do with about two hours less sleep per night and I've got a general sense of wellbeing which I never had before and clearer thinking/perception.'[3] Researchers commented, 'eating less than average by restricting calorie intake lowered rates of cardiovascular disease and cancer, increased life expectancy and dramatically improved the quality of late life by reducing chronic disease.'[4]

The National Academy of Sciences Human Study

Researchers examined a group of elderly people who had been on a calorie-restricted diet for six years and found they had improved blood-fat profiles, lower fasting glucose and insulin levels, lower body fat and a reduced level of C-reactive protein (a measure of inflammation). They also had marked improvement in memory (far more than a group taking omega 3 pills) and a decreased risk of degenerative brain disease.[5] Eating less improves and strengthens the immune system[6] and is a constant theme when examining the eating patterns of healthy older people who are living free from disease.

> I never eat meat and avoid fried food, I've never smoked and I hardly ever drink, I get up at 4.30 to do the washing and the rest of the housework, I'm in bed well before 9 pm, I eat just about anything, but I draw the line at Western food.
>
> Eriko Maeda, Japanese 70-year-old, 2010[7]

The CALERIE Human Trial

The five year trial called CALERIE, which stands for Comprehensive Assessment of Long-term Effects of Restricted Intake of Energy, has already shown that eating less reduces insulin levels, core body temperature, energy expenditure and RNA and DNA damage.[8] The CALERIE trial also showed increased cellular resistance to stress proteins, improved triglyceride levels and improved liver function markers.[9] These are all strong indicators of health and longevity.

Cuba

Cuba is a very clear example of what eating less can do for disease rates across an entire country. Cuba is also perfect to study as it has excellent national health data from national surveys, cardiovascular studies, primary care chronic disease registries and vital statistics over three decades. This has enabled an international team of researchers from Spain, Cuba and the US to analyse and follow what happened to the weight, disease and death rates from coronary heart disease, stroke and diabetes from 1980–2013.[10] In 1990 the USSR collapsed, so suddenly there was no money and no food being exported to Cuba during the years spanning 1991–95. This resulted in nationwide food and petrol shortages.

People were forced to do four simple things:

1. Grow traditional, local, vegetation rich, plant-based wholefoods.
2. Improve the quality of food eaten (you cannot grow junk food such as hamburgers, no matter how many you plant).
3. Eat less overall because there was far less food available.
4. Walk or use a bike as there was no petrol for cars.

How did the imposed 'eat less food and eat better quality food' experience impact on the health of the nation? The change was immediate, staggering and life saving. The preventable modern lifestyle diseases that had been ravaging Cuba all declined dramatically.

1. Deaths from diabetes dropped by 50%.
2. Deaths from heart disease dropped by 34%.
3. There was an average weight loss of 5.5 kg.

So, what has happened to the health of the nation since 1996, once the imported and processed sugar- and animal-rich food supply resumed?

1. There has been an average weight gain of 9 kg.
2. Since 1995, Cuban obesity rates have tripled.
3. Diabetes rates have grown by 140%.
4. Death from diabetes has risen every year since 1995.
5. Deaths from coronary heart disease and strokes have soared to well above the 1995 rates and continue to grow each year.

Long healthy lives: case studies

Japan

Traditional Japanese eat significantly less than we do. Japanese women have an 86-year life expectancy and a 1.5% obesity rate, with very low levels of sickness, low medication and low disease. Many Western women have a life expectancy in the 70s, a 35% obesity rate, with the last 20 years of life (from their 50s), usually dominated by sickness, hospitals, pain, drugs and disease. Japan also has the world's lowest infant mortality rate.

A traditional Japanese diet consists of fresh, plant-based foods such as brown rice, local and seasonal vegetables, fermented soy products, pickles and fresh fish. They have a custom of serving up small portions of food on their plate. The Japanese adherence to Buddhism and Shintoism also helps to keep the population svelte because of resctrictions on eating meat.

In 2013, seven of the ten oldest people in the world were from Japan. Of the world's 64 oldest people, 22 come from Japan. Misao Okawa is 115 years old. She is from Osaka and held the title of oldest living person, as well as oldest living woman, as at July 2013. Misao was 102 years old when she fell and broke her leg. A few days afterwards she was found doing leg squats because she didn't want her body to 'get out of shape'. Misao is a true role model; we should emulate and learn from her.

Korea

One 'longevity village' in Korea bases its diet on fermented soy bean paste and seasoned vegetables.[11] Kim Jong-nyuh, an 85-year-old resident, says, 'We usually eat kimchi, spring greens and fish. We don't really eat beef and pork.' Korean centenarians claim eating more vegetables, eating less overall and not drinking alcohol as their main secrets. Asked to what they attribute their longevity, 70% said they never drink alcohol, 54% cited eating in moderation, and 67% said they eat a lot of vegetables.

> Not one of them [25 Hunza centenarians] showed a single
> sign of coronary heart disease, high blood pressure, or
> high cholesterol levels. They have 20/20 vision and no tooth
> decay. In a county of 30,000 people, there is no vascular,
> muscular, respiratory or bone disease.
>
> Dr Paul Dudley White, Cardiologist, *The American Heart Journal*, December 1964

The Pakistan Hunza

For centuries the Pakistan Hunza were cut off by 7000-metre Himalayan peaks from the outside world. They lived on a sparse menu of fresh vegetables (mostly spinach), apricots (the national dish), walnuts, mulberries, cherries, apples, peaches, pears, potatoes, onions, sweet potatoes, yams, radishes, carrots and chapati/buckwheat cakes with sprouted lentils and other legumes. They ate flaxseed or linseed in some form with every meal. Many reached 100+ years old. Their key to health was nutritious food and eating less. Today they are consuming a typical modern diet and all is changing. In the past the Hunza people would die from falling off cliffs or by accident. Now they are experiencing hypertension, heart attacks, stroke, diabetes, obesity and cancer.

Campodimele, Italy

In her cookbook *A Year in the Village of Eternity*, Tracey Lawson writes that '111 of the 671 people who call Campodimele home are between 75 and 98 years old and the average life expectancy is 95. People walk everywhere. Everyone tends gardens, orchards, vineyards and fields, and they keep chickens and goats. They cook from scratch and prepare food for winter. A staple dish is fresh potato and green bean salad with fresh parsley, a few cloves of garlic, lemon juice and a splash of olive oil. Time spent preparing good food is regarded as an investment in health and happiness.'

Sardinia, Italy

In Silanus, in the highlands of Sardinia, of the 17,865 people born between 1880 and 1900, 91 have lived to their 100th birthday, a rate more than twice the average for Italy. Around 220 of Sardinia's current 1.6 million people have reached the age of 100. Recent Sardinian 100-year-olds number around 1460 people. The northern Sardinian centenarian rate is between 10 and 20 Sardinians reaching 100 for every American centenarian.[12] In the remote Sardinian Nuoro province, 66 people were found who were 100 years or more of age. Usually you find four centenarian women to every man but, in Sardinia, you have 2:1. In central Sardinia the ratio is 1:1.[13] This rate is 10,800 centenarians per million people!

In one village, 16 men and 14 women born between 1876 and 1912 reached their hundredth birthdays.[14] Sardinian Quirno Demurtas, 96 years old at the time, had the arteries of a 50-year-old man when tested (low blood pressure + good cholesterol balance = longer life). Efisio Puddu, 102 years old at the time, said, 'I always led a moderate life. I never drank too much.' His grandson Fabio says, 'When my grandfather was young, he ate less and drank less.'

The Sardinian people eat mainly plant-based, organic, local vegetable foods such as fava beans, wholegrains, vegetables, artichokes, tomatoes, oranges, figs, apples, apricots, grapes, mastic oil and locally made red wine (consumed only with a meal[15]). They are remarkably slim, as they eat around 70% of what average Westerners do.[16] They eat meat once a week, if at all, and it is usually saved for special occasions. Their exercise is rigorous and daily. It is not unusual for a 90- or 100-year-old Sardinian to milk cows, cut wood and then tend to sheep. These centenarians eat 1800 to 2100 calories a day, which is 30–50% less than your average Western intake. Sadly, obesity rates have recently soared with the introduction of processed foods.

The world's oldest family

The Sardinian Melis siblings, who live in the community of Perdasdefogu, are the world's oldest family. They are 105, 99, 97, 93, 91, 89, 81 and, the baby of the family, a young 78! One of the siblings, Alfonso, says, 'We eat genuine food, meaning lots of minestrone and little meat and we are always working. Every free moment I have I am down at my vineyard or at the allotment where I grow beans, eggplant, peppers, and potatoes.' His sister Claudia says, 'You just keep working and you eat minestrone, beans, and potatoes.'[17] Researchers at the University of Sassari in Sardinia said the family's longevity is influenced by the seasonal fruits and vegetables, particularly pears, prunes, or plums, that they consumed as part of their healthy Mediterranean diet.[18]

The Vilcabamba Incas, Ecuador

The Vilcabambans eat a fresh, local plant-based wholefood diet that has approximately half the average Western calorie intake. Vilcabambans regularly live into their hundreds and they have near-zero levels of diabetes, heart disease, cancers and other lifestyle diseases. They eat a vegetarian diet of fresh vegetation, such as avocados, quinoa, sweet potatoes, fruit, seeds, nuts, wholegrains and beans, and rarely eat an egg or two. Studies of these people showed there was an absence of a hormone known as IGF-1, or insulin-like growth factor, in their blood. IGF-1 has been implicated as an accelerant of cancers and as a powerful regulator of metabolism. Researchers from the University of Hawaii have also found variants of the gene that lowers IGF-1 in long-lived Japanese-American men on the island of Oahu. IGF-1 levels in the body can be controlled through diet by eating a plant-based wholefood diet and cutting down or avoiding animal-based foods such as hamburgers, pizza, fried chicken or meats. Eating animal foods will raise IGF-1 levels.

Bama is located in the Bama Yao Autonomous County in Guangxi, China. Chinese and foreign researchers announced in January 2010 that there were 90 centenarians living in Bama, making 36 centenarians for every 100,000 people. This is five times the international average. The healthy old people of Bama eat just two meals a day; eating considerably less than we do at around 1500 calories daily. They eat a local, fresh, plant-based wholefood diet that is naturally nutrient-rich and yet low in protein, fat, and cholesterol. The basis of the diet is potatoes, pumpkin, bamboo shoots, yellow corn, beans, wholegrains, hemp seeds and, of course, the famous green tea.

As reported by www.chinagaze.com and *Epoch Times*, 30 August 2013.

... those who are long-lived do share common features, including a positive mental state and a lower than normal intake of calories.

Zhang Tiemei, Deputy Director, Beijing Institute of Geriatric Medicine, Beijing Hospital, China

China

In an attempt to deconstruct the secrets to long life, Professor Yang Zhimin, Vice President of the Guangdong Province Hospital for Traditional Chinese Medicine, led a research team and interviewed 128 centenarians in Guangzhou.[19] 'We wanted to find out what they have in common, or their secrets. While heredity is an undeniable factor, we found that it is largely *their own efforts to keep a healthy lifestyle that contributed to their long life.*'

Those interviewed were between 100 and 110, and lived mainly in the old city district of Guangzhou. Yang and her team shared some of their findings that included the following:

▶ 90% have three meals at regular times each day

- 90% walk as their most common daily exercise
- 84% do not smoke
- 70% stop eating before they are completely full
- 68% do not drink alcohol
- 63% sleep at least eight hours every day
- 60% live with their families
- fresh fruits and vegetables are the most commonly eaten foods
- fatty and processed food is shunned and avoided.

A typical example is Xu Yuanshu, who at 110 years old eats a simple, plant-based wholefood diet of sweet potatoes and vegetables.

Based on these survey results, a low-calorie plant-based wholefood diet, regular healthy lifestyle habits, exercise, and an affinity for hard work can be considered keys to longevity.

From 1958–62, China experienced a great famine and millions of people were without enough food. Now, the biggest health problem in China is obesity. Throughout China, fast food is easy to find; there are simply too many people eating too much of the wrong sorts of foods. In 2013, nearly every street corner in Beijing and many other cities has a McDonalds or KFC outlet. Pizza Hut is (sadly) considered a 'fancy date night' restaurant. Coca Cola is sold at every corner stand, on every street. The WHO has found that overweight and obese Chinese adults rose from 7% in 1982 to 40% in 2012 of a population of 1.37 billion.[20] The perception of 'fatness' is still not understood in China. A 2012 Penn State study of 176 Chinese children aged 6–18 found that 72% of mothers of overweight children thought their children were 'normal or underweight'.[21] Our perception of a healthy size has changed as the human race has become fatter.

Hainan province, south China

Chengmai is a group of villages on the tropical southern island province of Hainan, China. This population group of elderly Chinese villagers is renowned, and they are reported to be one of the oldest groups of people on earth. Within the population of 560,000 people are more than 200 centenarians and at least three known supercentenarians (those aged between 110 and 120). This ratio is incredible given there are only around 400 supercentenarians in the world, and puts Hainan's people among the highest in the world. Experts who have studied these people say it's a combination of lifestyle habits promoted by the healthy environment.

> ... the lifespans of these residents are a result of a combination of a diligent, simple-minded and magnanimous lifestyle as well as mainly taking a vegetarian diet, and the classic 'early to bed, early to rise' ...
>
> Study sponsored by Chengmai's Communist Party Committee, August 2013

> There is not a lot of industry, the climate is good, they can get exercise easily, and the diet is healthy; they have plenty of fresh fruit and vegetables, and the soil is also naturally high in selenium.
>
> Jennifer Holdaway, Head of the China Environment and Health Initiative of the Social Science Research Council, visited Chengmai in 2012, as reported August 2013 by ibtimes.com

Dan, a good friend of mine, travelled through Thailand in August 2013. On his return home he sent me an email that I thought summed it up rather well. He said, 'The Thai people eat tiny portions, mainly vegetables, have squatting public toilets [very good for bowel health], walk and cycle everywhere, and don't seem to even know what dairy is ... can't think why they live longer though. Only logical conclusion is that they are genetically superior from birth.' He was, of course, being sarcastic when he wrote the last line!

France

French people avoided obesity and heart problems by eating a diet with a higher mix of fresh, highly nutritional foods as well as eating 25% less than their American counterparts. The average restaurant portion in the US was 346 grams; in France it was 277 grams. In supermarkets, 14 of 17 products sampled were up to 82% bigger in the US. However, today the 'French women are slim' illusion is waning. Child obesity is rising and the myth that French people can eat anything and stay thin is fading. Why? They are eating American-style fast foods in American 'supersized' portions.

Young French people are commonly eating anywhere, any time, and drinking out of large bottles of soda/cola/fizzy/soft/sugar-laden drinks. French women are getting fat, as are women in other European countries. Over 15% of French women are now clinically obese, with a further 26% overweight (41% total now overweight). Obesity rates have doubled in 15 years to reach seven million. French obesity levels (in the 18–24 age group) have grown 35% in three years. There are 22 million overweight French adults. Does this sound like a slim society? No. French men are the same, with recent statistics indicating 14% are obese and 39% are overweight (53% overweight). Between 1997 and 2009, the average French person put on 3.1 kg and added a further 4.7 cm around the waist. Not slim anymore.

Is wine the answer?

No, this is a total myth.

▶ Alcohol kills 49,000 French people each year (134 each day).

▶ Seven million people in France have a drinking problem.

▶ 13% of all male deaths are due to alcohol (one in seven).

▶ 40% of these alcohol deaths are young people under 65.

▶ Other results are cirrhosis, suicide and mental illness.

Does this sound like a healthy relationship with alcohol? Is this something to emulate? Good for the body and mind? Nope. The only small benefits of quality red wine are flavonoids and polyphenols, and these can be found in much larger amounts in fresh fruit and vegetables. The studies telling you that alcohol is good for you are bogus and are generally funded by the global alcohol industry.

> In France, alcohol is responsible for 25% of 15–34 age deaths.
> The causes of death attributable to alcohol are above all
> cancers and all heart diseases.
> Catherine Hill, Biostatistics & Epidemiology, Institute Gustave-Roussy, Paris, 2012

The island of Kitava, Trobriand Islands, Papua New Guinea

This population is characterised by extreme leanness and low blood pressure, with undetectable levels of heart disease, stroke or obesity. These people are healthy, with good skin and strong teeth. They eat less than we do and live on vegetables, tubers, fruit, fish and coconut. They do not eat dairy products, red meat, refined fat, sugar or breakfast cereals, nor do they smoke cigarettes or drink alcohol.

> They often say they prefer to eat only fruits and vegetables.
> Maurizio Berardelli, a geriatrician, 2013, on studying Italian centenarians

The Nicoya Peninsula, Costa Rica

The Nicoya Peninsula is a 120-kilometre slice of paradise, where the Pacific Ocean meets the tropical rainforest. In his book *The Blue Zones*, Dan Beuttner introduces the peninsula as another renowned place of longevity. Costa Rican men are known to enjoy particularly long lives, with an average life expectancy of 82 (at age 60). However, the elderly Nicoyans live two to three years longer than any other Costa Rican group. They live a traditional, agricultural lifestyle, eating a plant-based local wholefood diet and they eat *considerably* less than we do.[22]

The Seventh Day Adventists of Loma Linda, California

For over 30 years, researchers including the National Institutes of Health (NIH) have studied over 100,000 Californian Loma Linda Adventists to assess their life expectancy and risk of heart disease and cancer.[23]

Loma Linda is a vegetarian community. There are no liquor stores and the community has been legally smokefree for nearly three decades. *National Geographic* called Loma Linda 'one of the world's four blue zones' and 'the single healthiest place to live in America.' The average Adventist lives up to ten years longer than the average Californian, making them America's Centenarian Champions. They have ten centenarians per one in other US states.[24] How do they do it? Firstly, they eat significantly less than your average person. They eat a plant-based wholefood diet of beans, soy milk, tofu, mixed green salad, tomatoes, nuts, wholegrain bread and legumes, and drink at least five glasses of water a day. They eat no meat. They are fit, lean, smokefree, caffeine free and teetotal vegetarians.

Adventist Marge Jetton turned 100 in September 2004 and renewed her driver's license for another five years. She received the Philanthropist of the Year Award from a civic group at age 101. On a typical morning she power walked a mile at a good pace, lifted weights, rode her bike and ate her oatmeal. She lived to 106, and her tips were given as she tapped her perfect teeth: 'Exercise, eat wisely, love people and have a good attitude. I haven't eaten meat in 50 years, and I never eat between meals.'

Gary E. Fraser and colleagues from Loma Linda University led the Adventist Health Study-2, involving nearly 100,000 US and Canadian citizens.[25] The researchers reported that these strict vegetarians are, on average:

- 13 kg lighter than meat eaters

- 5 units lighter on the BMI scale

- live an average of 9.5 years longer

- have lower systolic and diastolic blood pressure and less hypertension (the number one cause of worldwide death is high blood pressure).

> If you're born in the year 2000 and the current trends continue unchecked, you will have a one in three chance of developing type II diabetes. We worry this will be the first generation of Americans who don't live as long as their parents did.
>
> Dr John E. Anderson, Vice President of Medicine and Science, American Diabetes Association

The Mediterranean diet

The Mediterranean diet is the most studied diet in history, with hundreds of independent scientific reports carried out on how it extends life and lowers diseases. The Seven Countries Study, published in 1970, found that Greek people closely following the Mediterranean diet had lower rates of cardiovascular disease, cancer and overall mortality than the other six countries in the study (USA, Finland, the Netherlands, Italy, the former Yugoslavia and Japan). Since 1970, the results of 'a healthier heart, lower cholesterol and blood pressure, lower cancer rates and up to 70% lowered risk of early death' have been repeated and confirmed in 1995, 2001, 2009, 2010 and 2011, in over 70 studies on more than 2.5 million people.[26]

The 'healthy' Mediterranean diet

The 'healthy' Mediterranean diet is the one followed in Crete and on the island of Ikaria in Greece. It is made up of a high intake of vegetables, legumes, wholegrains, fruits, nuts, seeds, olives, olive oil, herbs, spices and fish, and a near-zero intake of alcohol, meat and commercial dairy products. This diet improves liver health.[27] Improved liver health alone extends lifespan (for example, 95% of organ cancer patients die of liver failure).

Greek women have the lowest early death rates in the world: just 38 deaths per 1000 women before the age of 60.[28] In 2012, the oldest woman in the world was 120-year-old Miriam Amash, who is still living in Israel. She says the secrets to her extraordinary longevity are ingesting a great deal of olive oil, avoiding alcohol and eating lots of vegetables and herbs. Joan Riudavets Moll from Spain ate a healthy, fresh traditional Mediterranean diet and lived to 114 years old.

Longevity and the 'healthy' Mediterranean diet

The secrets of the Mediterranean diet seem to be the mixture of healthy nutritional compounds alongside smart lifestyle choices and habits. Researchers found that, simply put, 'those who most closely followed the healthy Mediterranean diet had lower disease rates and mortality rates and lived longer, healthier lives.'[29] The Mediterranean diet even counteracts a genetic risk of stroke.[30]

> Our study is the first to identify a gene-diet interaction affecting stroke in a nutrition intervention trial carried out over a number of years in thousands of men and women. The PREDIMED study design provides us with stronger results than we have ever had before. With the ability to analyze the relationship between diet, genetics and life-threatening cardiac events, we can begin to think seriously about ... making meaningful changes to the way they eat. Being on the Mediterranean diet reduced the number of strokes in people with two copies of the variant [gene]. The food they ate appeared to eliminate any increased stroke susceptibility, putting put them on an even playing field with people with one or no copies of the variant.

José M. Ordovás, PhD, senior author, Director of the Nutrition and Genomics Laboratory, USDA HNRCA, Tufts University, USA, August 2013

> We saw that the Mediterranean diet appeared to compensate for genetic influence.

Dolores Corella, PhD, scientist, CIBER Fisiopatología de la Obesidad y Nutrición, and the Genetic and Molecular Epidemiology Unit at the University of Valencia, Spain, August 2013

The island of Ikaria, Greece

Nearly 30% of all Ikarians live into their 90s. They have 50% lower rates of heart disease than average Greeks, 20% less cancer and zero cases of dementia. Ikarians not only live a long time, they also live well. They party hard, have sex into their 90s, walk hills daily (they walk everywhere), are very active, sleep whenever tired, have low levels of stress and eat significantly less than we do. They also fast regularly.

> Never eat food fried with butter, always sleep well and
> with the window open; avoid eating too much meat
> and drink herb tea – mint or sage.
>
> Kostas Sponsas, Ikaria, 100 years old

The Ikarians eat a vegetable-based, nutrient dense diet with plenty of greens and olive oil. Their diet is based around fresh vegetables, wild greens, beans, potatoes, fermented sourdough bread, legumes and tea, and is very high in extra-virgin olive oil and antioxidant rich fruits grown in their highly fertile mineral rich soil.[31] A typical Ikarian lunch is almost always beans, potatoes, greens and local seasonal vegetables. Ikaria boasts access to more than 150 vegetable varieties.

On average, Ikarians eat meat just five times a month, and that's only if it is available. They eat very little sugar and consume very little cow's milk, tending goats and drinking fresh milk from these animals. They eat what I consider to be the best version of the 'healthy' Mediterranean diet.

The Ikaria Study

Dr Christina Chrysohoou, a cardiologist at the University of Athens Medical School, conducted 'The Ikaria Study'. Looking at this and the information gleaned from the Harvard School of Public Health study of 23,000 Greek adults.[32] The Ikarian diet featured:

▶ low overall calorie intake

▶ large amounts of locally grown vegetables and wild greens (fennel, dandelion or mountain greens, spinach-like horta, and other wild plants such as kritamo and andrakla which are extremely high in longevity protecting plantioxidants)

▶ lots of beans (full of protein and fibre)

▶ lots of locally picked herb tea ('mountain tea' made from local herbs: oregano, sage, thyme, wild marjoram, mint and dandelion)

▶ lots of local extra-virgin olive oil (olive oil is a superfood and the only natural vegetable plant oil that can be harvested and extracted without chemical solvents and additives)

▶ potatoes

▶ fermented sourdough bread

- legumes

- vitamin-rich locally grown fruits

- fish twice a week

- meat only a handful of times per month (only 5% of total calories)

- home-grown food in mineral rich soil

- home-made goat's milk (the goats being milked by hand).

One interesting discovery made by Chrysohoou was that 80% of Ikarian males between the ages of 65 and 100 were still having sexual relations! This is the polar opposite of a typical Western male eating a typical Western diet and experiencing erectile problems in his 50s.

The science

A 2013 analysis of more than 1.5 million healthy adults using the 'healthy' Mediterranean diet showed a severely reduced incidence of cancer, cancer mortality, Parkinson's and Alzheimer's diseases.[33] The 'healthy' Mediterranean diet cuts cancer cell growth.[34] Those eating the healthy Mediterranean diet with more than three servings of nuts per week had a significant 39% lower all-cause mortality risk of early death, cancer or heart disease, compared to those not eating nuts.[35]

> The Mediterranean diet may be recommended for
> effective management of ... cardiovascular disease.
>
> Caroline Richard, registered dietitian and doctoral candidate
> in nutrition, Laval University, Quebec, Canada

The 'healthy' Mediterranean diet and weight loss

The 'healthy' Mediterranean diet may be among the most effective for promoting weight loss and diabetes management through diet. Dr Olubukola Ajala, a diabetes specialist at Western Sussex Hospitals in the UK, with her colleagues reviewed ten years' research covering 20 studies.[36] They compared the effect of seven popular diets on adults with type II diabetes. After following the diet for at least six months, the plant-based wholefood 'healthy' Mediterranean diet was the most effective for promoting weight loss and lowering blood sugar levels among diabetics; it improved heart health with 'good' cholesterol rising by 4–10% and triglycerides falling by up to 9%.

Heart disease and stroke

A group of men with major risk factors for heart disease and stroke ate the Standard American Diet of low fibre foods, high in meat, sugar and added fats, and then changed to a 'healthy' Mediterranean diet of high fibre foods, vegetables, fruits, wholegrains, legumes, nuts, seeds and olive oil. The 'healthy' Mediterranean diet lowered their 'bad' LDL cholesterol by 9% in just five weeks.[37]

In the work I do in thelifeplan, I have seen people's blood-pressure and cholesterol readings lower fairly easily and quickly when they switch to a recommended plant-based wholefood diet. The National Institute for Heath and Care Excellence (NICE) has issued new guidelines for all heart attack survivors to prevent further heart disease. The guidelines advise they 'eat a plant-based wholefood diet, eat more plants, lay off butter, cheese and meat, exercise every day, while fish can be eaten twice per week.'[38]

> People who have had a heart attack have a greatly increased
> risk of another. People who have had a heart attack should
> be encouraged to eat a healthier, Mediterranean-style
> diet, and exercise daily in order to reduce their risk of
> a further heart attack.
>
> Professor Mark Baker, Director of the Centre for Clinical Practice at NICE, UK

Memory and brain health

The 'healthy' Mediterranean diet can lower your odds of chronic kidney disease by 42%.[39] Those who most consistently ate the 'healthy' Mediterranean diet were 13% less likely to develop memory and thinking problems, and those who ate more olive oil and omega-3 fatty acids and avoided red meats, dairy and cheese were 19% less likely to have cognitive problems.[40] The 'healthy' Mediterranean diet, heavy on extra-virgin olive oil and nuts, does more to keep the aging brain agile than simply switching to a diet without these natural oils.[41]

A plant-based wholefood diet

In one study, the 'healthy' Mediterranean diet benefits were, 'meta-analysed[42] from 41 prospective cohort studies on nearly three million people. According to the cumulative analysis 17% of the benefits come from low consumption of meat and meat products, 16% from high vegetable consumption, 11% from high fruit and nut consumption, 11% from high monounsaturated to saturated lipid ratio (largely due to olive oil consumption), and 10% from high legume consumption.'

A changing diet

Unfortunately, the Greek people are turning away from their traditional 'healthy' Mediterranean diet in large numbers, trading their incredible variety of fresh, local, healthy foods and lower calorie intake for a modern diet and a much higher calorie intake.[43] Of seven European countries in 2010,[44] Greece had the highest rates of obese and overweight children, with 20% of all 10–12 year-olds categorised as obese, and a further 30% overweight. The Greek obesity rate for children is now 40% and rising. This is not genetic, but is caused by decisions to change from a plant-based wholefood diet to the disastrous Standard American Diet (SAD) and lifestyle.

> It has to do with many factors. In the fifties and sixties the people were poor, but they were healthy. They were eating very good foods; olive oil, olives, the green leafy vegetables that are our treasure.
>
> Christina Makratzaki, Greek, Crete-based dietitian

> World trade has opened up a world marketplace in food that's like nothing the world had ever seen before. Nearly every society is going through what Crete has gone through – even in places where hunger is still endemic. It's known as 'the nutrition transition'. The nutrition transition happens very quickly. As soon as people get money, they start buying more meat and more processed foods. Well, that's fine if you don't eat too much of it. The problem is that we as humans, when we're confronted with large amounts of delicious food, we eat large amounts of food.
>
> Marion Nestle, New York University nutritionist

Longevity and centenarians

The Calabrian centenarians, Italy

A study on centenarians in Calabria showed that 'the genetic component of longevity appears to be stronger in males, but women may take better advantage of external factors such as diet and medical care than men do.'[45] This confirms the old cliché that women look after themselves better than men. Most of us know this to be true. The Calabrian centenarians tended to possess a particular gene important to taste, allowing them to enjoy bitter foods such as broccoli and field greens. They ate far more of these than most people and it helped them to live longer. This is obviously and easily controllable through diet; simply eat more bitter greens.

The Ashkenazi centenarians, New York

The Einstein Project, which studied more than 500 centenarians in and around New York City, found that the Ashkenazi centenarians have exceptionally high levels of HDL, often called the 'good' form of cholesterol.

The Taiwanese centenarians

In Taiwan, the Jinhu and Jinning townships in Kinmen County, Shuangxi District in New Taipei City, Shihtan Township in Maioli County, Jiangjyun District in Tainan, and Fonglin Township in Hualien County all have populations of over 10,000, where many people have reached the age of 90 and above. These elders are physically active and eat the fresh, local, seasonal vegetables and fruits that they have grown themselves.

Eating less

As you age, your body tissue accumulates collagen fibers and becomes stiffer. When you weigh less, the heart is happier, stronger and more relaxed. This alone keeps you younger for longer and enables you to exercise regularly, bringing many other benefits. Weight loss by eating less (and helped by exercise) restores some of the heart's youthful elasticity.[46] This makes it easier for the heart to relax between contractions and refill with blood.

In 2010 Gary Fagg, at 60 years old, had a near-perfect body mass index (BMI) of 20. In 2007 he hiked down the north rim of the Grand Canyon and up south rim hill – nearly 102 km, 21 of which were straight up. Gary is over six feet tall and eats around 2300 calories daily. He eats less and has all the energy he needs.

> We were quite surprised by the Mediterranean diet in particular.
> I would have thought that low-carb would have been the best
> for losing weight, but Mediterranean seems to be better.
>
> Dr Olubukola Ajala, UK

Longevity is strongly linked to food, calorie intake and exercise habits, far more than genetic and environmental factors such as where you are born, who your parents are or what your genes are. Lower calorie and super-healthy diets with daily physical activity are the secrets for extended lifespans with minimal incidence of diseases such as high blood pressure, heart disease, cancer, diabetes, rheumatism, osteoporosis, Alzheimer's and vision problems.

The Abkhasian National Geographic Studies, 1970s

Dr Alexander Leaf, a Professor of Clinical Medicine at Harvard University and Chief of Medical Services at Massachusetts General Hospital, studied the people of the Caucasus mountainous region of Abkhasia (pronounced ab-car-zha) in Southern Russia, and wrote about his study in a series for *National Geographic* magazine. Dr Leaf studied health and habits, and took blood pressures and blood tests. He was staggered by the health of these elderly people. They were without heart disease, cancer, obesity, diabetes and all the other preventable diseases we take for granted as we age. He found many extremely elderly locals with a healthy blood pressure of 118/60 and cholesterol levels of 98. Remember, the biggest cause of death in the world is high blood pressure and heart disease. Not in Abkhasia!

Dr Leaf found 80% of all Abkhasians over the age of 90 were mentally well, healthy and outgoing, while only 10% had poor hearing and less than 4% had poor eyesight. Can you imagine what our world would look like with 80% of our 90-year-olds in such exceptional health? They had very low stress levels, did things at their own pace, walked everywhere and moved all day long.

Dr Sula Benet, a professor of anthropology, also lived and studied these wonderful people. In her book, *Abkhasians: The Long-Living People of the Caucasus*, she said, 'sickness is not considered a normal or natural event, even in very old age.'

The Abkhasians usually eat a breakfast that includes a salad of freshly picked wild green vegetables, such as tomatos, cabbage, cucumbers, watercress, green onions, radishes and onions, with a porridge and a warm, fermented drink. They also eat lots of nuts for the protein, and good fats. They are basically vegetarians, as they eat very little meat. Most of their meals are raw or mostly raw, without added oil, butter or salt. They eat an enormously high amount of fruit, all locally grown and picked fresh. There is fresh fruit available year round: apples, pears, apricots, cherries, figs, plums, peaches, persimmons and berries of all kinds. When there is nothing fresh, they eat fruit they have preserved naturally. They eat less than 2000 calories per day, which is around half of the average in Western countries.

Healthy at 100

In his book, *Healthy at 100*, John Robbins did a fantastic analysis that compared the calorie intake, food choices and overall diets of the Abkhasia, Hunza and Vilcabama people to see if they had any similarities.

What he found was stunning. Three of the world's longest-lived peoples, in the best health, with the lowest disease rates, ate the same basic intake of macronutrients. Much more interesting is that they all got their nutrition through plants. Here is how he compared them.

Food Intake	Abkhasia	Vilcabamba	Hunza	Average*
Calories from carbohydrates (vegetables, wholegrains etc.)	65%	74%	73%	71%
Calories from fat	20%	15%	17%	17%
Calories from protein	15%	11%	10%	12%
Overall daily calories for men	1900	1800	1900	1866
Plant foods as a % of diet	90%	99%	99%	96%
Animal foods (including dairy) as a % of diet	10%	1%	1%	4%
Salt intake	low	low	low	low
Sugar intake	0%	0%	0%	0%
Processed refined food intake	0%	0%	0%	0%
Incidence of obesity	0%	0%	0%	0%

* I have added in an average score to show the basic overview of food intake

What can we learn?

The longest-lived and healthiest centenarian populations around the world (including the Okinawans of Japan) all do the same thing: they eat a plant-based wholefood diet of vegetables, fruits, nuts, seeds, wholegrains and legumes, with very little meat or dairy foods.

They eat around half the calories of the average Western diet: 1800 calories daily.

They move every day; it's a normal part of their day.

They have no obesity, diabetes, cancers, heart disease and all the other preventable illnesses that are killing 70–95% of us.

Amy Tombs (1906–2011) is an example of how eating less promotes premium health. Through my beautiful and inspirational Granny Amy, I saw how effective eating less and eating well, combined with daily

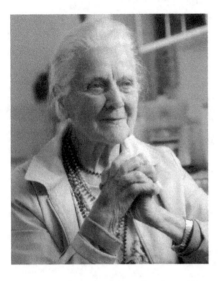

movement, could be. When I visited her in England in 2005 (she was 99) she greeted me with a big hug, asked if I was hungry, and then went outside to her garden, picked some fresh vegetables, and made me a delicious fresh salad. We sat, ate and talked for three hours. She was as sharp as a pin and engaging in all manner of topics about life and the world.

Amy was an inspiring, gentle, warm, gracious, intelligent, well-informed, wise old woman. She was a mentor to me. When it was time to go, she walked me to the bus stop. She was the absolute blueprint of how I want to be when I get older: healthy, with a sharp brain, a wonderful sense of humour and the ability to spend time with grandchildren and great-grandchildren and be

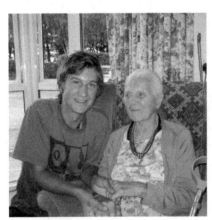

Trey with Amy, his great-grandmother, August 2010.

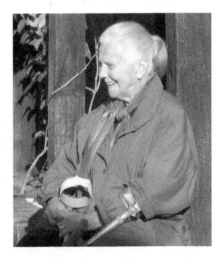

engaged with them. In August 2010 my eldest son, Trey, spent three days sitting and talking with her. He said, 'Dad, I see what you mean about Amy, she is just magical!'

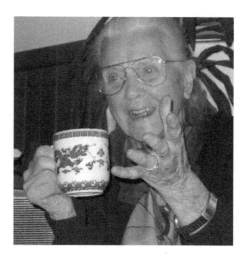

On her 103rd birthday we had a great old chat and she told me she 'had no illness of any sort, my heart is fine, though my eyesight is deteriorating and I wobble now when I walk!' It is mind blowing to think that she was only ten years away from being the oldest person alive on the planet!

Granny Amy was a strict vegetarian for the last 81 years of her life. She became a vegetarian (near-vegan) in 1930, at the age of 23. She told me in February 2010 that she does have a splash of cow's milk in a cup of tea, saying, 'I wish I were a vegan, I just don't like the taste of soy milk!' Because Granny Amy was my step-grandmother, I can't count on any 'longevity genes' to get me to 100-plus in good health. However, she was always my darling Granny Amy and her legacy to me is her inspiration.

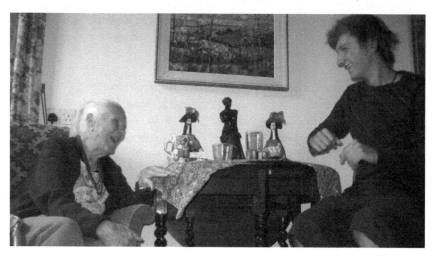

Okinawa, Japan

The single most impressive and overwhelming evidence that health and longevity come from eating a local, fresh, plant-based wholefood diet and eating far less than we do is demonstrated in the 161 beautiful islands of Okinawa, Japan. The elderly people on these islands have been studied very extensively. In Okinawa, every village, town, island and city has meticulously recorded birth and death records reaching back to 1879.

After 30 years of exacting study by medical research teams from the Okinawa Centenarian Study and The Okinawa Program, it was concluded that the three leading killers in the West, heart disease, stroke and cancer, occur in elderly Okinawans with the lowest frequency of any population studied by modern science. By 1995, Okinawan life expectancy had surpassed the absolute limits of population life expectancy estimated by the Japan Population Research Institute and many biodemographers.[47]

Okinawa is home to the world's healthiest documented elders, to the world's longest recorded life expectancies, and to the highest concentrations of verified centenarians in the world.

John Robbins, author, USA

The Okinawans boast the world's longest life expectancy, the world's healthiest lifespan and the world's highest count of centenarians. They also have around 15% of the world's verified super-centenarians (aged 110 and older), despite a relatively small population of 1.4 million residents! This is less than 1% of 1% of the world's population. They do all of this in great health, with energy and mobility, and with the lowest rates of heart disease, stroke and cancer in any elders anywhere in the world.

The Okinawans have a low risk of arteriosclerosis and stomach cancer and a very low risk of hormone dependent cancers, such as breast and prostate cancer. They eat more tofu than anyone else in the world ... they eat as low down the food chain as possible.

Dr Craig Willcox, American gerontologist,
co-author of The Okinawa Program

The Okinawa Centenarian Study

The Okinawa Centernarian Study started in 1976.[48] The population of 1.4 million has over 670 people living into their second centuries, mostly very active and looking decades younger than their actual age. Interestingly, around 90% of their centenarians are women. This is a common theme around the world.

Elderly Okinawans have impressively young and clean arteries, and low cholesterol and low homocysteine levels when compared to Westerners. These factors reduce their risk for heart disease and stroke by up to 80%. Male Okinawan elders are 88% less likely to die from prostate cancer, while women are 70% less likely to die from ovarian cancer and 70% are less likely to die from colon cancer than average. The Centenarian Study has consistently found that lifestyle, rather than genetics, is the major player in keeping Okinawans healthy for life. At the heart of the Okinawan lifestyle is their cultural habit of 'hara hachi bu', which means 'to stop eating when you are 80% full'. The Okinawan people experience a healthy, vital, disease-free and drug-free long life on a daily intake of around 1800 calories. This is half our typical, modern average of 3500 calories.

The Okinawan diet is a plant-based wholefood diet, rich in sweet potatoes, much like the 'healthy' Mediterranean diet. They do not eat processed fatty foods or polished white rice, or drink cola drinks. They do not overeat, smoke cigarettes or drink coffee or alcohol. They do not eat meat, except for very rare ceremonial occasions. They eat traditionally prepared soybean dishes like tofu, natto and miso soup; sweet potatoes called imo and konnyaku; many servings of wholegrains such as brown rice; mugwort (an aromatic plant), seaweed, onions, broccoli, nuts, seeds, wholegrains, tomatoes, kudzu (a legume), bitter melon, bamboo shoots, pickles and flaxseed. They eat fish (dried bonito) two or three times per week. All of this is garnished with garlic, ginger and turmeric, and washed down with copious jasmine and green tea!

The secret to a long healthy life? Even the doctors ask me that question. I think one thing is the diet. I tell people when they're too heavy that they should reduce some of the weight.

Walter Breuning, 114, the world's oldest man
on 31 August 2010

Soy foods

The Okinawans eat more soy foods than any other group on earth, consuming between 60 and 120 grams of soy per day. They eat eight times more tofu than the Western average. They eat natto, a fermented soybean dish in large amounts. Natto is a rare and particularly abundant vitamin K source that helps protect against fractures, osteoporosis and bone degenerative diseases. Naturally processed soybean superfoods such as tofu, tempeh, edamame, miso, tamari, soymilk and natto have shown strong evidence of reducing cancer risks. This was confirmed in the Okinawa Centenarian Study.[49] The researchers concluded that high soy consumption is one of the main reasons that Okinawans are at extremely low risk for hormone dependent cancers, including cancers of the breast, prostate, ovaries and colon. The lowest cancer rates in the world are found in the Okinawans.

Okinawans live a basic 'let your food be your medicine and your medicine be your food' preventative health approach, integrating much of what is good about Eastern medicine with the best of the West. They enjoy gentle and daily physical activity in the form of dance, martial arts, gardening and walking. Moving your body every day is very important, as the more time you spend sitting and not exercising, the faster you die.[50] The Okinawans do not sit all day, they move regularly and they live the longest. They do not have high rates of smoking, but they have strong social and community support for the elderly. In the traditional language there is no word for 'retirement'.

The Okinawa Fountain of Youth[51]

► The Okinawans eat 34% vegetables, 32% wholegrains, 12% soybean foods, 11% fish, 6% fruit and barely 5% dairy foods or meats. Their diet is the exact opposite of our modern processed sugar- and meat-rich diet.

► The Okinawans have the highest rate of people living to 100–120 years old.

► Over 97% of the population is disability free. This is the longest disability-free life expectancy in the world.

► There are almost 700 centenarians per million people, seven times higher than in other populations in the West.

► Obesity and diabetes levels are the lowest in the developed world.

► Okinawans have 17% of the heart disease rates of Americans and are far less likely to suffer coronary heart disease, strokes or cancer.

► Okinawans get colon cancer at half the rate of those in other Western countries.

► Breast, ovarian and prostate cancer all occur at 20% of the rate of others in the West.

► Okinawans have 33% less dementia than Americans.

► The negative experience of menopause is an unheard-of phenomenon.

One hypothesis is that the secret about ageing is to avoid accumulating molecular damage, and eating fish, beans, nuts, seeds, legumes, whole grains, and not so much red meat, dairy or sugar may help us to reduce that kind of cellular damage. In the early days we did try to link health with specific foods or nutrients, but now we look more holistically at dietary patterns.

Professor John Mather, Director of the Institute for Ageing and Health at Newcastle University, UK

The centenarian researchers found that the Okinawa diet leads to:[52]

► finely tuned digestive tracts due to the smaller amount of food, and the diet being raw, fresh and prebiotic-nutrient-enzyme-rich

► low cardiovascular risk owing to diet, exercise and a relaxed attitude; elderly Okinawans have clean arteries and low homocysteine levels, meaning their hearts are stronger, fitter and healthier

► low cancer, obesity and diabetes rates due to the high fibre fruit and vegetable intake, abundance of good oils, and low body-fat levels

► strong bones due to a physical life spent under the natural sunlight and a diet favouring vitamin C-rich vegetables and fermented foods

► very mild menopause symptoms due to a high intake of natural oestrogens from soybean foods and flax.

Japan has the best longevity statistics in the world and Okinawa is home to the oldest, healthiest people.[53] Even the world's oldest dog, Pusuke, was Japanese! We can learn a great deal from these humble, community-minded people. They have the highest number of centenarians and the longest 'healthy life expectancy' without requiring drugs, and without getting the diseases that kill Westerners at relatively young ages.

In May 2010,[54] Kama Chinen, from Okinawa, was the world's oldest person.

> I don't drink or smoke; I work in my garden, ride my bicycle
> and go for walks. Keep close to your friends and
> don't worry because stress kills.
>
> Katsu Yamakawa, age 95, best friend of 114-year-old Kama Chinen.
> Katsu eats lightly cooked fish, seaweed and rice, fresh fruit, vegetables,
> and her 'miracle food' goya (a bitter melon), and drinks green tea.
> As reported by Reuters, AAP and stuff.co.nz, 30 August 2013.

As at July 2013, the oldest person in the world was 115-year-old Misao Okawa, from Okinawa. Sadly, the next generation of young Okinawans have changed their dietary habits. They are consuming Western foods such as hamburgers, pork and cola drinks in record amounts, and they are now suffering increased rates of illness.

Sadly, it is often the people who eat less and live long that complain about not having enough food and they look to the US and Europe as signifying prosperity, satisfaction or happiness. However, we have seen that Western food habits cause a long, slow, health decline peppered with pain, physical problems, medication and early death. This is nothing to aspire to; rather we should take inspiration from the traditional Okinawan lifestyle. However, Okinawan life expectancy has now started to decline; this can partly be explained by the change to a modern, Western diet.

> Never in the history of nutrition research has the evidence been
> more clear and consistent: a high 'wholefood carbohydrate, low
> calorie, plant-based diet' is the best for long-term health. There's
> no doubt about it anymore, despite what you might have read in
> books advocating low-carb, high-animal-protein diets.
>
> The Okinawa Centenarian Study Researchers in 2010, after 37 years of meticulously
> following the healthiest, oldest and longest-lived population in history

8
Processed foods + overeating + overweight + obesity = short lifespan

People who survive to at least 100 years tend to be lean and not have diabetes or diseased arteries.

Nobuyoshi Hirose, Director of Geriatric Medicine, Keio University, Tokyo

The exportation of Supersize Me

Japanese people are now also eating Western-style foods in record amounts. Western takeaway restaurants are prolific. American 'supersize' meals are becoming the norm. A 2009 study by the European Congress on Obesity concluded that increased energy intake was the most significant cause of the rise in obesity in the US since the 1970s. This fatness and obesity has now hit every Western-influenced nation on earth, including Japan.

Caution: American-size portions served here.

Sign in a Hong Kong restaurant window, August 2009

Weight gain

As waistlines expand, so does the perception of a healthy weight. The 'fat is okay' trend is avoiding the ugly truth that weight gain is the number one factor causing Western disease. There are no fat centenarians. Every study on long-term weight gain concurs that you will die younger and have much higher risk of NCDs by being overweight. The first and most important hallmark for longevity is staying in healthy, lean shape. The heavier and more overweight you are, the higher your chances are of suffering strokes, cancer, heart disease, diabetes, osteoporosis, arthritis, mental disorders and dying young.

In all parts of the world, people are getting fatter. In 2006, 60% of Western men and 50% of Western women sampled were either overweight or obese, compared with just 7% in Eastern Asia.[1] Western women are gaining on average 650 grams each year, this is the extra 10 kg that sneaks on every decade or so.[2] It has become socially acceptable to be fat, simply due to the number of people that are. Over 60% of overweight and obese people surveyed believe that their body weight (and that their overweight or obese children) fell in the acceptable range and that this would still let them live a long, healthy life.[3]

People underestimate how much bigger we all are because so many of us are overweight. We see so many large people now that we think being anything less than very large is fine. Our perception of size has changed – and grown. Due to the sheer number of overweight people, we now embrace being overweight as 'their right' (which of course it is) and we are trying to make being overweight okay and acceptable.

I actually agree with this philosophy, as it is your right to be the shape and size you wish to be. However, this does not change what being overweight will do to your health and lifespan. Nobody is talking about the fact that being overweight will result in more time and money spent at the doctor's and the hospital, or that it dramatically and immediately raises your risk of all the preventable killer diseases such as cancer, diabetes and heart disease, or that it will shorten your life by up to 60 years.

A shortened life

Obese men in their 20s are twice as likely to die by age 50, and are up to eight times more likely to suffer a heart attack, a fatal blood clot or diabetes, than their lean counterparts. They are three times more likely to get any of these serious conditions than their normal weight peers by middle age.[4] We are now expected to die at a younger age due to the extra weight we are carrying. Longevity is slowing thanks to the high calorie diet and processed foods we are eating in record amounts. Men in their 30s are 20% more likely to be overweight than in previous generations, and women in their 20s are twice as likely to be obese.[5] Young people are now more likely to get high blood pressure, obesity, cancer and diabetes than their parents ever were. Being overweight or obese is likely to shorten your life by at least 10–15 years.[6] The more overweight you are, the shorter your life.[7]

It is important that people realise that obesity in a young age is a serious risk to long-term health. The effect obesity has on cardiovascular death has a greater impact in younger age groups. Young adulthood obesity also increases the risk for premature death among women. Obesity related morbidity and mortality will, in decades to come, place an unprecedented burden on healthcare systems worldwide.

Dr Morton Schmidt and Henrik Toft Sorenson, Department of Clinical Epidemiology, Aarhus University Hospital, Denmark

A reality check

Being overweight or fat, or carrying a large waist, contributes to over 50% of fatal heart attacks and gives men up to a 180% increased risk of heart failure. When overweight, the fat cells around your stomach operate as an active organ that sends 20 hormone and chemical signals to other parts of the body.[8] These chemical messengers increase the risk of heart attacks, cancer and other diseases. Being overweight raises the ovarian cancer risk for women by 80%[9]. It causes 24% of adult onset diabetes, 24% of osteoarthritis, 22% of cardiovascular diseases, and 20% of colorectal, breast, uterine and kidney cancer,[10] and accelerates the growth of many cancers by more than 50%. Being overweight from an early age boosts the risk of premature death by 50%,[11] causes weaker bones and osteoporosis,[12] and gives an 80% lower chance of reaching age 70 without disease.[13]

Being overweight causes excess fat around your waist to coat your organs; even a small deposit of this fat increases your risk of serious health problems.

Adrian Bauman, Professor of Public Health, University of Sydney, Australia

In 2008, over 124,000 people in Europe developed cancer through being overweight.[14] Being overweight will become the biggest cause of cancer deaths in women by 2016. A large belly gives an 80–360% higher chance of developing Alzheimer's or dementia,[15] gives women more than double the risk of dying of heart disease, stroke or cancer,[16] and dramatically increases your risk of dying young.[17]

Being overweight gives a 180% higher risk of suffering or dying of breast cancer,[18] increases your risk of painful fibromyalgia by 60%,[19] and leads to sexual problems such as low libido for women and impotence for men.[20] The more overweight you are, the smaller and more aged your brain becomes,[21] and the faster your reasoning, memory and other mental skills deteriorate.[22]

Overeating while pregnant leads to obese babies with a higher risk of diabetes.[23] The daughters of obese mothers are far more likely to be overweight.[24] Almost 50% of stillborn babies or babies who die in the first weeks of life have mothers who are overweight or obese, which supports the theory that the weight of a mother can be recognised as an attributing factor in infant mortality. Children born to overweight mothers have more body fat, live a much shorter life, and have up to 50% higher risk of congenital heart defects, other illnesses and early death.[25]

Being overweight in your 40s dramatically increases the risk of multiple chronic diseases, impaired cognitive function, loss of physical function and mental health in your 60s.[26] The more overweight you are, the more medications and drugs you take as you are more prone to chronic illness.[27] Being obese at 40 years of age means a life expectancy of 68, while at 20 years of age it means you lose 13–20 years of life.[28]

Children and weight

As a kid, being obese doubles the risk of heart disease and early death.[29] The heart problems we saw 20 years ago occurring only in the elderly are now seen in obese teenagers worldwide.[30] Obese children also suffer leg pain, deformed skeletons and aching bones from carrying excess weight.[31]

Overweight and obese children are developing the ailments of their grandparents. A 5 year-old weighing 60 kg or a 10 year-old hitting 100 kg are experiencing the typical modern elderly health conditions: hypertension, high cholesterol, type II diabetes, joint problems, fatty liver disease, sleep apnea, asthma, gallstones and gastroesophageal reflux. Over 60% of obese youths have high blood pressure, high cholesterol or unhealthy blood sugar levels (and usually a combination of all three).[32]

Obesity and cancer

Being overweight or obese is directly linked to some of the toughest cancers to treat: breast, cervical, ovarian, colon and rectal, endometrial, esophageal, thyroid, gall bladder, kidney and pancreatic cancers. Being overweight or obese also means a higher recurrence of cancer and lower mortality rates.

Those who became obese between the ages of 14 and 19 have a 100% increased risk of pancreatic cancer.[33]

Obesity significantly increases colorectal cancer.[34] Obese children have 50% higher risk of colon cancer than children of normal weight.[35] Obesity gives men a 57% increased risk of developing prostate cancer.[36] Obese people have a 21% higher risk of dying from cancers of the large intestine, breast, ovary, cervix and prostate, as well as leukaemia.[37] Those with the highest 'waist-to-hip' and 'waist-to-height' ratio are 2.5 times as likely as those in the lowest tertile to be diagnosed with liver cancer. Even a small increase in waist-to-hip and waist-to-height ratio is correlated with a 56% higher risk of gall bladder cancer.[38] Obesity raises the risk of renal cancer by 48%.[39] A bigger belly gives a 43% greater risk of cancer overall.[40]

> Obesity is a major risk factor for developing cancer, roughly the equivalent of tobacco use, and both are potentially reversible. Further, obese cancer patients do worse in surgery, with radiation or on chemotherapy; worse by any measure.
>
> Dr Karen Basen-Engquist, PhD, Director of the Center for Energy Balance in Cancer Prevention and Survivorship, and Professor of Behavioral Science, University of Texas, USA

Obesity, heart disease and strokes

Obesity doubles your risk of kidney stones,[41] and directly leads to diabetes, hypertension (high blood pressure, the number one cause of death in the world) and strokes.[42] A bigger belly gives a 44% greater risk of cardiovascular disease.[43] Severely obese infants have heart-disease risk factors as early as age two.[44] The longer you are overweight, the more dangerous your condition becomes. After age 50, excess body fat hardens the arteries, increasing your risk of dying from all aspects of heart disease, from heart attacks to high blood pressure to cardiovascular disease.[45]

Other health risks

▶ You are at a massive 85% increased risk of asthma if you are an obese woman.[46] For every increase in body mass, the asthma risk is shown to increase by 6% among women and 3% among men.[47]

▶ Overweight or obese children and teenagers have four times the risk of gall bladder disease.[48]

▶ Being obese and eating a poor quality diet are both directly associated with pre-kidney disease.[49]

▶ Men diagnosed with attention deficit/hyperactivity disorder (ADHD) as children are twice as likely to be obese.[50]

▶ Fertility rates have been dropping steadily for 100 years all across the Western world. Obese men aged 14–20 have up to 50% less total testosterone than do normal males of the same age.[51] This significantly increases their potential to be impotent and infertile as adults and to suffer type II diabetes.

▶ Being obese shortens your cell chromosomes, telomere length; the shorter your telomere, the higher your risk of high blood pressure and early death.[52]

Results support the hypothesis of a master plan, based on subtle intervention, that has been developed by the food industry to instil doubt regarding the adverse effects of sugar sweetened beverages and to prevent the implementation of public health interventions and policies aiming to reduce their consumption.

Dr Philippe De Wals, PhD, Laval University, Quebec City,
at the European Congress on Obesity in Liverpool, May 2013

The situation has reached crisis point and people must be made aware that excess fat will affect their immune systems and therefore their survival.

Associate Professor Katherine Samaras, Garvan Institute of Medical Research, Sydney

Weight loss is important, but so is nutrient quality.

Katherine Zeratsky, registered dietitian, The Mayo Clinic, Minnesota, USA

Our current system for assessing calories is wrong.

Richard Wrangham, evolutionary biologist, Harvard University, USA

The food you eat has an enormous impact on the gut bacteria, and, in turn, on the energetics of digestion. Bacteria in the gut respond differently to processed foods.

Rachel Carmody, evolutionary biologist, Harvard University,
from her studies of the energetics of digestion, USA

Net caloric counts for many foods are flawed because they did not take into account the energy used to digest food; the bite oral and gut bacteria took out of various foods; or the properties of different foods themselves [such as fibre content], that sped up or slowed down their journey through the intestines, such as whether they were cooked or resistant to digestion.

Food researchers, *ScienceNOW*, 21 February 2013

Soda pop is a quintessential junk food. It's just pure calories, and no nutrients. It's like a bomb in our diet. And let's not forget that soda has been linked to heart attacks, diabetes and osteoporosis, too.

Michael Jacobson, Center for Science in Public Interest, USA

The West is in the midst of an obesity epidemic and counting calories has been misleading. The quality of calories is as important as the quantity of calories. Sweetened drinks are the only specific food that clinical research has directly linked to weight gain.

Dr David Ludwig, paediatric endocrinologist, Boston Children's Hospital and Harvard Medical School, USA

A calorie is a calorie. There is no scientific evidence that connects sugary beverages to obesity.[53]

Katie Bayne, President of Sparkling Beverages, Coca Cola US, 2012

Efforts by industry elements to obscure the link between soda and health outcomes are in the interests of shareholders, but certainly not the public health. Whether or not the beverage industry has a coordinated master plan to obscure the association between soda and obesity, they certainly are motivated to downplay the importance of the relationship.

Dr David L. Katz, Yale University, USA

Where's the truth?

When you read the previous quotes from scientists, food researchers and evolutionary biologists, I am sure you can make a discerning observation about who has our best health interests at heart. I vote for those trying to tell us that it is the quality, type, preparation, style and amount of food that we eat that makes the biggest difference, not the drink company trying to sell us their synthetic sugar water.

Drawing overwhelming evidence from a myriad of sources, I believe the studies and the experts saying that being overweight or obese is healthy are fundamentally flawed, as are food or drink companies trying to tell you their 'constipating, fatty, sugar-filled, acidic, synthetic products' are healthy.[54] They are not, they never have been, nor will they ever be.

Is a calorie a neutral thing?

Think about it. Take two genetically identical twins. Say one twin ate 2000 calories per day for three months, garnered from only breakfast cereals, hamburgers, fries and cola drinks. The other twin ate 2000 calories per day for three months, garnered from only fresh fruits, vegetables, legumes, wholegrains, nuts, seeds and water. After three months their blood pressure, heart-disease markers, cholesterol, body weight, weight circumference, fat levels, pre-diabetic and metabolic syndrome markers, and nutritional levels are all tested.

The twin who consumed breakfast cereals, hamburgers, fries and cola drinks would be irritable, carrying more fat and constipated, and with higher blood pressure, worse cholesterol balance and much lower levels of all the micronutrients and macronutrients.[55] This twin's health profile would show how sugar calories decimate the human system.

The twin who consumed fresh fruits, vegetables, legumes, wholegrains, nuts, seeds and water would be flying high, feeling great, with better skin, bowel motions, energy levels and heart health, and less body fat. This twin would also be emotionally different: calmer and happier.

A calorie is a calorie? These genetically identical twins would have changed their genetic expression by way of their diet and this would take them in different directions. When you digest food, different balances of gut microbiota alter the rate of calorie absorption during digestion. These differences are overseen by the interaction between the quality and amount of food you eat and your gut.

So, the argument that 'a calorie is a calorie, no matter where it comes from' is at best weak and can be repudiated easily, regardless of how it is sold or how many times it is repeated to us in advertising.

> Collectively, the studies all support the view that restriction of the consumption of sweetened drinks will facilitate weight reduction. Given the scientific evidence presented in these and other articles, restriction of high-caloric sugar-laden beverages would be one simple measure to stem the tide of the growing obesity epidemic.
>
> Gerard Mullin, MD, MHS, Johns Hopkins School of Medicine, USA

Soft drinks and obesity

There are many studies that show soft drinks cause obesity and help you become overweight. Doctor Sonia Caprio of Yale University wrote in the *New England Journal of Medicine* that, 'calories from sugar-sweetened beverages do matter'.[56] The University of Sydney, in a study of 2000 12 year-olds, found that the children who drank one or more soft drinks each day had increased risk of heart disease and high blood pressure.[57] A Boston Children's Hospital study examined 224 overweight adolescents for 12 months and found that children who drank sugary soft drinks gained twice as much weight[58] as their counterparts. A University of Adelaide study on 16,907 people found those drinking many soft drinks were 79% more likely to have a respiratory disease.[59] Consuming sugary drinks affects the genes that regulate weight and increase – the genetic predisposition of a person to gain weight – so avoid them if you are interested in healthy genetic expression and a lean strong body.[60]

Swapping water to take up calorie laden, synthetic, high sugar, junk food drinks that go down easily is deadly. These drinks include not only your obvious sugary sodas, but those of the 'vitamin water, smart water, nutrient water' variety as well. They claim to be healthy, but there can be enough sugar in a 500-millilitre bottle to provide the average person with a third of their recommended daily intake. You can consume more calories in one small junk-food feast than in the rest of the meals in the day combined. Drinking calorie filled, nutrient sapping, junk food sugar drinks is aging you, sip by sip, wrinkle by wrinkle.

A latte on your way to work, a can of cola with lunch, a juice before the gym and a beer after work can together add an extra 700 calories to your daily energy intake. High fat content in cow's milk and larger cups means the coffee you buy can contain well over 500 calories. That's 25% of your daily calorie requirement in one highly processed, adrenal exhausting, acidic drink.

Also to note is that the negative effects of junk foods that produce damaging inflammatory changes are longer lasting in the obese and overweight.[61] Again, you can be caught in a vicious, biochemical, food addiction cycle of sugar, salt, fat and gluten that directly leads to inflammation and weight gain.

Two-thirds of the calories in the average Western diet come via anti-nutrients, that suck nutrition out of the body, cause acidity and premature aging, and provide zero health benefits. This leaves one-third of the diet to provide enough nutrients for general health, to make up for the nutrient-deficient foods we are eating, to create the enzymes required to break the anti-nutrient foods down and to combat pollution, stress, toxins and pesticides.

Your waist measurement and your weight

Having a large waist means large amounts of visceral fat around the abdominal organs, which can cause inflammation, high cholesterol, insulin resistance and other problems linked with poor health. As previously discussed, a thickening waist is a risk factor for heart disease, cancer, respiratory failure and early death.[62]

Can you lose it? Yes. A 16th-century Italian nobleman, Luigi Cornaro, was very overweight and seriously ill by age 45. Told to eat less, he became one of the first people to write extensively about the benefits of food restriction. Cornaro voluntarily restricted his food intake and lived to 102, an extraordinary achievement for the time (he lived from 1464 to 1566).

Over 7000 studies (including by the World Cancer Research Fund) tell us that being even slightly overweight increases the risk of cancer of the oesophagus, liver, pancreas, bowel, breast, kidney, prostate, ovary and womb. Over 90,000 needless cancer deaths per year could be avoided if we ate less.

In one study, after six months of eating less, 48 middle-aged, overweight men and women all showed a significant decline in DNA damage.[63] The results showed that a significant reduction in food intake caused a reversal in DNA fragmentation, with decreased insulin levels and core body temperature. These are three biomarkers of longevity. Their bodies changed how they used energy when less food was offered. The basic theory is that you have less energy going in; therefore the body produces less, causing less damage.

So, eat less, eat well and live long!

9
A plant-based wholefood diet
+ Regular Intelligent Fasting®
= a long healthy life

> Over 70% of our health outcomes are predicted by our behaviors and our environment.
>
> Laura Jackson, Wellmark Insurance Company, USA

It is always encouraging to see scientific proof that it is the little things you do each day that affect how long and healthy your life is going to be. A massive study, from which the above quote comes, called 'Does overall diet in midlife predict future aging phenotypes? A cohort study', was published in May 2013 in *The American Journal of Medicine*. It clearly confirms that aging and health is all about diet and lifestyle.[1]

The study found that a plant-based wholefood diet was significantly associated with low risk of heart disease or early death. Results included information about the negative effects of eating a typical modern, processed, sugar-rich and meat-rich diet. Consumers of such a diet:

► were 50% less likely to reach old age

► were 50% less likely to age without disease

► had a 53% greater chance of cardiovascular death

► had a 36% greater chance of non-cardiovascular death

► had poorer musculoskeletal status (weak bones)

► had worse cognitive function (a weak and forgetful mind).

We showed that specific dietary recommendations may be useful in reducing the risk of unhealthy aging, while avoidance of the Western-type foods actually might improve the possibility of achieving older ages free of chronic disease and remaining highly functional.

Low adherence to healthy diet and lifestyle recommendations is associated with increased premature death and the Western-type diet significantly reduced the likelihood of achieving ideal health at older ages ... independent of other health behaviors such as physical activity and smoking.

Dr Tasnime Akbaraly, PhD, and colleagues, INSERM, France, in the *American Journal of Medicine*, May 2013

Four key behaviours

The multi-centre 'Multi-Ethnic Study of Atherosclerosis' (MESA), a long-term and ongoing prospective examination of the risk factors, prevalence and prevention of cardiovascular disease found four behaviours that together wipe out about 80% of the chance of getting heart disease.[2]

Lead author Dr Haitham Ahmed, at the Ciccarone Center for the Prevention of Heart Disease, John Hopkins University, said in June 2013, 'To our knowledge, this is the first study to find a protective association between low-risk lifestyle factors and early signs of vascular disease, coronary heart disease and death, in a single longitudinal evaluation. Those who adopted all four healthy behaviors had an 80% lower death rate over that time period compared to participants with none of the healthy behaviors.'

The four key behaviours are:

▶ not smoking

▶ eating a healthy, balanced, plant-based, wholefood diet

▶ getting to a healthy weight and maintaining it

▶ regular exercise.

Piet van den Brandt, Professor of Epidemiology at Maastricht University, did an analysis of a 25-year international study on 120,000 people. He said that 'Few studies worldwide have analysed the relationship between lifestyle and mortality.' Researchers found that those who did not smoke, moved regularly, ate a plant-based wholefood diet, and kept themselves at a healthy weight 'lived around 15 years longer and the benefits were regardless of age'. The 1976–2012 Nurses' Health Study is one of the most comprehensive diet/lifestyle/mortality studies ever done. It found the most protective health behaviour was simply 'eating more vegetable fibre.' The 1950–2012 International Adventist Health Study of almost 100,000 people found that 'eating a plant-based wholefood diet extends longevity by ten years'. Another research project, 'Successful prevention of non-communicable diseases: 25 years' experience with North Karelia Project in Finland', found 'a plant-based wholefood diet gave an 80% drop in heart disease mortality, a reduction in all mortality by 45% and greater life expectancy by seven years.'

Scientists at the Max Planck Institute for Demographic Research in Germany, in 2006, confirmed longevity is not a genetic trait.

The World Preservation Foundation (WPF) did a meta-analysis of studies and research and said, '75% of common chronic diseases such as cancer, obesity, diabetes and heart disease could be eliminated if people simply ate a wholefood, plant-based diet.'

The more fruits and vegetables consumed in a state, the lower it is on the obesity rankings.

Trust for America's Health and Robert Wood Johnson Foundation, 2012

Diabetes

A 2011 study conducted by the National Heart, Lung, and Blood Institute at the National Institutes of Health on 200,000 people found five habits that made the biggest difference to diabetes risk:

▶ eating a plant-based wholefood diet

▶ maintaining a healthy weight

▶ not smoking

▶ low or zero alcohol intake

▶ regular exercise.

The results did not vary for those who had a family history of diabetes or were overweight. Family history and genetics had nothing to do with it. These five lifestyle factors cut the type II diabetes risk by 80%.[3]

Epidemiologist Jared Reis, PhD, and lead author of the study, said, 'We found that for each factor added, the risk of developing diabetes was lowered. There is a clear benefit in adopting all five.'

A healthy weight

At my largest, I weighed 80 kg. This may not seem very heavy, but on my small frame, believe me, I was porky pants, as my friend Dave told me. I changed to a plant-based wholefood diet, eating less and moving daily with smart lifestyle changes, and lost nearly 20% of my weight in this healthy sustainable way. I am now the lean and healthy 70 kg I was as a teenager. Over time simple, daily changes bring the biggest results.

Your body fat levels shift upwards over time, at around 500 grams every few weeks, if you are constantly overeating or eating the wrong sorts of foods. The truth about real, long-term and healthy weight loss is that it takes time and effort. To reset your body metabolism you must commit to hard work for at least a year. This changes your future, and the sooner you start, the less disease you will suffer and the longer your life expectancy. To shift your body fat down you do it slowly, otherwise your body will cannibalise your muscle, excite your fat storage enzymes and give you a ravenous appetite.

You don't need to 'pack it on' as you get older. Improve your diet. Eating around 2000 calories of the right foods daily helps the brain recover better from injury and fight degeneration, and is the best longevity ingredient in your recipe for life.[4] Even a small weight loss is enough to change and improve your immune cells and reduce damaging inflammatory cells by 80%. We know that long-term inflammation leads to all the killer diseases.[5]

Cutting sugar

In a study on worms, restricting sugar in their food set off a process that extended the lifespan of some worms by up to 25% (the equivalent of 15 human years). Without sugar, the worms' physiology altered and they quickly built up better defences, became stronger and lived longer.[6]

Cutting all sugars and sugar substitutes out of your diet will help you live longer[7] and lower your risk of cancer.[8] In many ways, sugar directly causes cancer,[9] inflammation being one of the effects of sugar. It has been found that excess sugar in the modern diet feeds cancer growth.[10]

There are plenty of natural sugars in fruits and vegetables. Natural sugars such as glucosamine protect your joints. These beneficial sugars can be damaged by stress, leading to crippling conditions such as osteoarthritis. However, consuming too much processed sugar causes our bodies to produce excessive amounts of insulin, which means the level of sugar in the blood can suddenly crash. This can cause incredible hunger. You then eat more and feel hungry again soon afterwards, and the cycle keeps going. Foods high in processed sugars are usually very low in nutrition. When the body's nutritional needs are not met, it continues to crave food, hoping it will get some nutrition, which again explains the non-stop eating. The more refined sugars you eat, the fatter you become, the higher your cancer risk, yet the more malnourished you actually are. It is a vicious and dangerous cycle.

Why are we overweight?

Nobody wants to be fat. Overweight and obese people say they would give up a year of their life rather than be fat. Up to 30% said they would rather walk away from their marriage, give up the possibility of having children, be depressed or become alcoholic than be obese.[11]

The good news is that you can lose weight. Neither the number of your fat cells nor their size is genetically fixed.[12] You are not born fat (unless you have an obese mother). It takes years of overeating to grow fat.[13] Remember, genetics are not to blame for obese or overweight children. Children become obese because of their diet, lifestyle and environment and the influence of their parents.[14] Solely due to poor diet, obese mums are ten times more likely to have obese daughters. Obese dads are six times more likely to have an obese son.[15] At least 30% of teenagers are now at risk of coronary disease due to weight-gain and inactivity.[16] Obesity at 20 means you are twice as likely to die young of a preventable disease.[17]

10
Weight-loss drugs and weight-loss surgery

In 20 years 60% of the world's adult population could be overweight. It's not regional, it's global, it's increasing rapidly, it's continuing to escalate – the basic definitions of a pandemic.

Linda Fried, Mailman School of Public Health, Columbia University, USA

The global 'Weight Loss Management Market' was worth US$265 billion in the year 2012 and is expected to grow to US$361 billion by 2017.[1] If we stay overweight, we benefit the weight-loss industry, potentially becoming life-long customers as we continue to buy their 'new and improved' product, be it a pill, a lotion, a drug or a service.

The weight-loss management market has within it three distinct sectors: diets, services, and fitness and surgical equipment. The weight-loss diets market includes weight-loss foods, drinks and pills. Weight-loss food is the largest segment of the weight-loss diets market and contains dubious 'foods' such as meal replacements, low calorie ready meals, sugar free confectioneries and low calorie desserts. I do not recommend you look at any of these foods as a solution to your weight problem. Remember, a lot of people are making an enormous amount of money, but making no difference to the people they are supposedly helping. The focus must be on what goes in the mouth, alongside an exercise routine.

Eating a plant-based wholefood diet will have you shed your excess weight in a healthy, long-term and sustainable way. Do not be fooled by high protein = weight-loss diets. The Laplanders, Greenlanders and the Russian

Kurgi tribes have the highest meat-protein consumption in the world. They are also among the populations with the lowest life expectancies, often dying when they are barely 30 years old. Inuit Greenlanders, with very limited access to fruit and vegetables, have the worst longevity statistics in North America, usually dying about ten years younger and with a higher rate of cancer than its neighbouring Canadian population.

Japan has 37 centenarians per 100,000 people. Canada has less than half that, at 17 per 100,000. The WHO predicts a total of 3.2 million centenarians by 2050, with over 30% of them being Japanese. That is one small country having a third of all the oldest people alive in the world.

Hundreds of studies, over hundreds of years, looking at centenarians and people of all ages, races, creeds, colours, body types, blood types and sizes in countries all over the world, have shown that the more meat you eat, the more weight you gain, the sicker you become, and the more you are at risk of heart disease, cancer, obesity, diabetes and early death.[2]

> Selling anti-obesity drugs over the counter
> will perpetuate the myth that obesity
> can be fixed simply by popping a pill.
>
> Dr Gareth Williams, University of Bristol, UK

High protein, animal-rich diets

High protein, animal-rich diets encourage weight gain due to the damage they do to the body, and the focus on animal foods displacing vegetables. Animal foods lack the fibre, carotenoids, plantioxidants and essential nutrients that you get only from vegetables. Even the leanest beef is still a whopping 29% saturated fat. Skinless chicken is still 23% saturated fat. Take 140 grams of chicken and you get a measly 40 grams of protein. When you cook meat you lose another 50% of the protein, so that 140 grams of chicken actually gives you a tiny 20 grams of usable protein (which your body then has to break up before it can be used). If you fry the chicken, you are adding more dangerous trans- fats. As a comparison, vegetables are generally barely 5% fat and these are the good, protected, essential fatty acids, not the bad fats. Good fats are in plentiful amounts in healthy superfoods such as seeds, nuts, avocados, coconuts, olive oil and green vegetables.

Weight-loss drugs and weight-loss surgery do not work long term

Many studies have shown that after four years, most people using weight-loss drugs are back to their original weight. The side effects of weight-loss drugs include high blood pressure, heart attacks, cancer, strokes, liver damage, digestive problems, uncontrolled bowel movements, bloating, insomnia, nausea, depression, memory loss, mood disorders, anxiety, birth defects and even death.[3] These side effects exactly mirror statistics showing health conditions that are killing around 90% of people in the West.

If you choose to have gastric banding, do your homework beforehand. Understand that you need dramatically to change the way you eat after the surgery for it to be successful, as most body fat returns within a year.[4]

In a massive review of over 50 different studies on weight-loss surgery, long-term follow-ups found those who had weight-loss surgery often did not maintain their loss.[5] Risks of surgery are serious and include bleeding, infection, slippage of the band, blockage of the stomach outlet or nutrient loss, leading to osteoporosis and anaemia. People have also died during and after surgery.[6]

Gut bacteria

As you lose weight, your gut changes and increases the health-promoting bacteriodetes population. Your gut bacteria run your immune system and most of your aging processes. Many people are subject to the vicious cycle of weight gain causing poor bacterial growth, causing ill-health and disease, causing weight gain. Changing the health of the gut bacteria will drive weight loss.[7] Weight loss can be driven by a plant-based wholefood diet.

The three dominant family groups of bacteria in the human gut are fimicutes, bacteriodetes and actinobacteria. To remain healthy with a strong immune system, you need a proper ratio between the fimicutes and the bacteriodetes. The more overweight you are, the higher your fimicutes. The leaner and healthier you are, the higher the bacteriodetes.[8]

In 2008, The National Institutes of Health Human Microbiome Project started funding varied 'Health and the Human Gut' studies around the world. So far they have discovered links between gut microorganisms and the development of influenza in young children, digestive disorders of all kinds, skin problems and cancer. The University of Maryland School of Medicine scientists identified standard communities of bacteria that were common to all. However, the people with high blood pressure, insulin resistance, metabolic syndrome and obesity also had 26 other rare intestinal bacteria linked to insulin resistance, high blood pressure, cholesterol imbalance and high blood sugar levels.[9]

A different diet means different bacteria

The single most powerful way to change the gut and the bacteria lining is by changing diet. Colon, gut, intestinal, bowel and digestive health are all reliant on your microbiome. Microbiota (gut flora, microbiome, healthy bacteria and so on) in lean, healthy people is different from that of unwell or obese people.

Healthy people have a higher proportion of bacteroidetes. A study in the *European Journal of Clinical Nutrition* in 2010 found the probiotic *lactobacillus* helped lower abdominal fat and body weight. In 2009, the *Journal of Gastrointestinal Surgery* reported greater weight loss among those with higher *lactobacillus acidophilus* probiotics. Studies in *Bioscience, Biotechnology, and Biochemistry* (2010) and *Obesity Research and Clinical Practice* (2008) found that probiotics improved weight loss.[10]

The prebiotic- and probiotic-rich superfoods that best transform our gut are the high fibre, whole plant foods such as fruits, vegetables, nuts, seeds, wholegrains and legumes, as well as natural fermented foods. The natural fibre-rich plant carbohydrates also protect the bowel from growing dangerous bacteria.[11]

Eating more plants will lead to healthier gut bacteria

Healthy rural African children eating a local, fresh, plant-based wholefood diet have a very different gut bacteria profile than overweight Western children. Diet influences gut bacteria more than any other single aspect of lifestyle. Plant-based wholefood diets have a direct and powerful effect on bowel health, pretty much the opposite of the modern sugar-rich and meat-rich processed diet.[12] Genetic expression in the gut is dominated by food interaction, and it is cleaned, fed and run by a plant-based wholefood diet.[13]

Low plant, high animal diets are deadly

A 25-year Swedish study has shown that high fat, low carbohydrate diets do not deliver long-term weight loss, do not lower your BMI and, in fact, do dramatically raise your risk of heart disease and death.[14] The study began in 1986, after concerns about the high incidence of heart disease in northern Sweden. Over the 25-year period there was no sign that high fat, high protein, low carbohydrate dieting of any kind helped people lose weight. The average body size showed a consistent rise in both men and women.

Professor Ingegerd Johansson, the leader of the study from the University of Umea, said, 'While low carbohydrate/high fat diets may help short-term weight loss, then results of this Swedish study demonstrate that long-term weight loss is not maintained.'

New Zealand is the world leader for bowel cancer

New Zealand women have the highest colon cancer rates in the world, and they also have the highest dietary intake of red meat (which contains no fibre).[15] New Zealand men have the world's third highest colon cancer rates. In most Western countries (including New Zealand), we eat a low fibre, highly processed, animal-rich diet. This is almost a guarantee for bowel disease.

Bowel cancer is the most frequently diagnosed cancer and the second-highest cause of cancer death in New Zealand. We are currently the world champions in bowel cancer rates. We eat one of the lowest fibre diets in the world. We have the highest bowel cancer rates. Bowel cancer kills over 1200 Kiwis and over 4000 Australians every year. This is three times the New Zealand road toll. It means 100 people per week, or 14 people every day, die from bowel cancer in New Zealand and Australia combined. The WHO, The Cancer Society and the World Cancer Research Fund have illustrated that bowel cancer is only 3% genetic. In essence, we lose 97 New Zealanders and Australians every week to bowel cancer. These people could still be alive if they ate a different diet and lived a different lifestyle. Saddest of all, bowel cancer numbers, incidence and death are growing in the 20–39 age groups faster than in any other group.

> Data from this large prospective study suggest that obesity is important throughout the natural history of colorectal cancer and colorectal cancer prevention efforts should encourage the achievement and maintenance of a healthy body weight.
>
> *Journal of Clinical Oncology*, May 2013

How do we reverse the disease rates?

Eating well and not being overweight lowers bowel cancer risk immediately. Being overweight and eating the modern diet raises the risk of bowel cancer immediately.[16] Vegetable fibre (found only in vegetables) is the most powerful bowel cleanser, regulator and protector we have. Obesity is associated with significantly increased risks for colorectal cancer.[17]

The average New Zealander has a very high bowel cancer and stomach cancer risk, due in part to following the Standard American Diet (SAD), which is rich in processed animal foods and sugar, and very low in vegetables.[18]

The GBD Study (2013) states that the fourth most prevalent cause of death on planet Earth is poor nutrition. Nearly one in three New Zealanders is eating themselves to an early grave by ingesting too much meat, chicken, sugar, processed foods and takeaways, and by not consuming enough fruit and vegetables.[19] If you eat less than five servings of fruit and vegetables daily, you have a 53% higher risk of dying compared to those who have consumed five servings a day.[20] This risk remains, regardless of other factors such as smoking, drinking and body weight.

Weight loss is 80% diet, 20% exercise

Weight-loss experts from all over the world have been very clear that weight loss is 80% diet and 20% exercise. As far back as 1932, obesity expert Russell Wilder said to the American College of Physicians, 'My patients lost more weight on bed rest than on an exercise regime.' The diet and lifestyle of the Hadza people of Tanzania has changed little in 10,000 years: they still live as hunter gatherers, so they are a great model of much older human diet and lifestyles. The people eat mostly vegetables, berries, roots and fruit, using digging sticks and axes, and sometimes getting lucky when hunting animals using bows. Researchers measured the energy expenditure in 30 Hadza men and women aged 18–75. The physical activity, exercise and movement of the Hadza was much higher than of people in modern societies, but when corrected for size and weight, their metabolic rate was no different.[21]

The researchers found that even among these ancient peoples, in their natural environment and eating their natural diet, the amount of calories we need is a fixed human characteristic. This clearly shows that we are growing overweight and obese through **overeating** rather than a **sedentary lifestyle**.

> One of the greatest marketing myths that the global fast food industry pulled off was to make people believe that losing weight is all about exercise and nothing to do with diet. The sheer brilliance of this lie moves all the attention away from what these companies put into the modern foods they sell...'
>
> Jason Shon Bennett

Brazil and America

According to Brazilian Health Ministry Data released in April 2012, more Brazilian people are exercising but more Brazilian people are overweight. This study of 54,144 people in Brazil's 27 different states found that 48% of Brazilians are overweight (up by 5.3% since 2006) and 16% are now obese (up by 4.4% since 2006), yet more people are exercising!

Over 63% of the key 35–45 age group are overweight. Sedentary males fell from 16% in 2009 to 14% in 2011. The really important part of the story that almost every single media organisation missed was that '80% of Brazilians do not even eat 5+ daily servings of fruits and vegetables anymore'.

It is the same in the US. Obesity rates are continuing to climb every six months despite more Americans exercising.[22] Even school exercise does not drop weight in children, unless they eat differently.[23]

Burn off junk foods by going for a jog!

No! The 'exercise = weight loss' idea was started in the 1980s with the explosion of television celebrity workout and aerobic shows. In one study in 2011, hundreds of women were assigned different amounts of exercise (or none) for a year. After 12 months all the women lost similar amounts of weight, regardless of exercise.[24] Weight loss is about smart diet and lifestyle choices, not just exercise.

Sleep

Sleep is critical to any weight loss or longevity effort. On average, New Zealand women sleep 6.5 hours per night. This is not even close to a healthy routine. Over 55% of Kiwis have sleeping problems, as we mostly undersleep.

Sleep affects your entire health profile, from weight, skin, energy, fertility and longevity to disease risk. Every 90 minutes of sleep you miss, you generally eat around 500 calories more. You know what I mean? Instead of going to bed at 9 or 10 p.m. and having a long, deep sleep, waking early to greet the day, what do we do? We stay up late, sitting and watching television, usually after sitting in the car or on the bus, sitting while working, sitting while eating an unhealthy high calorie lunch, and then sitting while eating dinner! Then what do we do? We sit some more while we watch television! At night we eat, and we eat the worst kinds of foods – pizza, hamburgers, chips, biscuits, lollies, alcohol and chocolate drinks – because sleepy people make bad food choices. Nathaniel Watson, a neurologist and Co-Director of the University of Washington Medicine Sleep Center in Seattle, and colleagues, analysed self-reported data on the height, weight and sleep duration of 604 pairs of identical twins and 484 sets of fraternal twins in the University of Washington Twin Registry.[25] They found that those who slept longer at night had lower BMI than those sleeping less. For those participants averaging more than nine hours of sleep, genetic factors accounted for 32% of weight variations. However, for those sleeping less than seven hours, genetic factors accounted for 70% of weight variations. Dr Watson commented, 'The less sleep you get, the more your genes contribute to how much you weigh. The more sleep you get, the less your genes determine how much you weigh.'

Cock crows in the morn to tell us to rise,
And he who lies late will never be wise,
For early to bed and early to rise,
Is the way to be healthy, wealthy and wise.

Attributed to Benjamin Franklin

What is the real culprit?

The Standard American Diet (SAD) is the main culprit. It is high in constipating animal foods, processed meats of all kinds, sugar-rich refined carbohydrates and the worst kinds of fats. Then it's washed down with acidic coffee and alcohol, in huge amounts. SAD has near-zero levels of plant fibre or real nutrition. Mix this toxic 'pretend food' with the modern highly stressed, rushing, low rest, no routine lifestyle and you have serious issues. Unless you are an elite athlete (they generally eat very well), and you are doing three or four hours of exercise daily, you cannot eat the modern diet and lose weight.

The simple truth is that eating too much, and eating the wrong sort of foods, destroys your gastrointestinal system and leads to weight problems. Weight problems lead to a sedentary life, which leads to more weight problems and tiredness and then craving the wrong sorts of high calorie junk foods. Here is that vicious cycle again.

People who achieve successful long-term weight-loss results change their lifestyles and habits, and eat very differently afterwards – otherwise the weight simply returns. Essentially, to lose weight you've got to change your relationship with lifestyle, sleep, stress, routine, food, exercise, movement and, mostly, what and how much you eat.

Thelifeplan is the best way I know to help you lose weight, get well and stay well. More information can be found at jasonshonbennett.com

11

Eat less, eat better, move more, have a rhythm, live long

Eating a third less than average, on a plant-based wholefood diet, and making smart lifestyle choices, is the best protection against disease, decline and poor health.

Jason Shon Bennett

How old is old? Is old the new young?

Over 30% of people would like to live past 90 and they have a real chance of doing so if they change to a healthy lifestyle.[1] The Western average is, at best, 100 centenarians per million people. In Okinawa, where they eat 30–50% less than Westerners do, they have over 700 centenarians per million people. Their most mentioned secret to longevity is simply 'eating less'.

Personally, I rate your stage of life from the human potential of 120 years. This means age 1–49 is young, 50–79 is middle-aged, 80–99 is elderly, 100+ is legendary, and those aged 110+ are The Super-Centenarian World Champions. As evidenced by the world's oldest people, the longest-lived people in good health, and the world champion centenarians, living long, healthy lives free of drugs and disease, your health is in your own hands.

My patients want to feel better, get back their energy, their libido.
People come in and have terrible diets, terrible lifestyles and they
want quick fixes. You have to do some lifestyle modifications.

Dr Richard A. Bligh, Medical Director, St Louis Center for
Preventive and Longevity Medicine, USA

Why is no one is pushing the 'eat less' message?

Why do you not hear about this everywhere? Why is this not shouted from the rooftops by doctors and health ministers everywhere? Simple: there is no money in it. No one will make money selling an idea like this, so no one is going to spend money educating the population on how to eat less. The food manufacturers will not like it, as less food will be bought. The pharmaceutical giants will not like it, as fewer people will get sick, so fewer drugs will be sold. The vitamin pill makers will not like it, as people will be healthier. If you eat less you become less of a consumer.

For starters, the benefits of a low calorie diet are low BMI, decreased cell damage and clean arteries.

Families would be healthier and parents would live longer, in better health. People would experience stronger, healthier and more satisfying lives. Joy and gratitude for what we have would grow. Equity and sharing would increase, as people realise that they don't need to stuff more in, they have more energy to give, and they can share more instead.

The focus could move to thriving, not just surviving. When you are vital and healthy, you have far more energy to help others. You are not just surviving your own illness.

> The toxic environment of Western diets causes hormonal imbalances that encourage overeating.
>
> Robert Lustig, MD, paediatrician, University of California, USA

Golden Rule No. 1: Eat Less

People are always asking me where I get my energy. Here's a supertip: eat less and get more (energy that is). It's amazing how 'leaving a little space for God' (as I heard someone put it so poetically) makes such a huge difference to your energy levels throughout the day. Practice *hara hatchi bu*. It means, 'Push yourself away from the table when you're three-quarters full.'

It is likely that the leaner you are, the longer you will live. You'll be giving the body exactly what it needs and not stressing it any more than need be. You have the total and utter power to influence your aging process every time you put something into your mouth.

It is not up to anyone else. It is up to you.

More than 33% of US centenarians who were questioned in a 2011 poll credited their longevity to good living. They said they had made a specific decision to eat well, limit alcohol, exercise regularly, manage stress in their lives and, of course, avoid smoking. Nearly 50% said the best advice they have is to 'spend more time with your families'. Dorothy de Low, aged 100, competed at the 15th World Veterans' Table Tennis Championships in Mongolia in 2010. The Hurstville great-grandmother was at her eleventh tournament since taking up table tennis at age 50.

Eating less lowers your risk of almost every disease as you age and the body changes the way it delivers your energy and vitality. Young Elvis was one of the most incredible looking, talented and vital young men of the 20th century. He died much too soon, aged 40; obese, depressed and drugged, after years of junk food that included fried banana and peanut butter sandwiches and greasy doughnuts. It does not matter the state of your health currently, or the age you are right now. Eating less, while maintaining a full nutritional intake, starts to heal your body immediately. You grow younger and healthier and you get sharper and more energetic every day.

> A quality breakfast, a light supper and eating to 70% full in
> three meals, are good preventative prescriptions to illnesses.
>
> Cao Yanjian, an established longevity expert during the Qing dynasty

The benefits of eating less are myriad. Many have been discussed so far; here are some of the main points.

▶ You get a reduction in visceral fat that leads to lower inflammation, which lessens your risk of obesity, diabetes, osteoporosis, cancer or heart disease.

▶ Your body responds to less energy input by activating enzymes that boost the rate of cellular repair and regeneration.

▶ You get an improvement in your immune system, limiting DNA damage and aging.

▶ You add between 20 and 30 years to your lifespan.

▶ You stimulate disease-preventing genes, while disease-promoting genes, including those involved in prostate and breast cancer, shut down.[2]

▶ Less energy is used for digestion, meaning less free radical damage.

▶ Your telomere cells are protected from aging, keeping your chromosomes stable. The longer the telomere, the younger and healthier you are.[3]

▶ Improved mitochondria function (the energy you have at a cellular level).

- You make better food choices.

- Stimulates your 'longevity gene'.

- Lowers three biomarkers of longevity: fasting insulin level, core body temperature and DNA fragmentation.

- Slows your metabolism, meaning less free radical damage.

- Changes the 'use of energy' the body works on. Basically, the body is not worn out by the action of constant metabolism. Less energy coming in means less energy being used and created, therefore less wear and tear.

- Stimulates the proteins that are responsible for increasing lifespan.[4]

> Diet, well-ordered, bears the greatest part
> in the prolongation of life.
>
> Francis Bacon

Tips for success when eating less

- Eat only when you are hungry.

- Eat a plant-based wholefood diet. This means reducing or eliminating animal foods such as meat and dairy. (See thelifeplan for more on this.)

- Eat three meals per day, well spaced out and planned in advance.

- Eat a soaked home-made muesli, full of healthy nuts and seeds, for breakfast for a sustained energy boost that will last until lunchtime.

- Instead of nibbling on food between meals, drink water.

- If you 'just gotta eat' between meals, eat raw fruit or vegetables.

- Eat slowly – you will not eat as much as you would eating at pace.

- Eat raw, sprouted, fermented, soaked, steamed and cooked foods.

- Start using smaller plates and bowls.

- Participate in the JSB life-changing 12-month health mentoring programme called thelifeplan.

- Swap coffee for a healthy variety of herbal and green teas.

- Don't be fooled by advertising for any of the fast food so-called restaurants. It is all a treat, nice once in a while, but not healthy.

- Eat more high fibre foods such as vegetables, fruits, nuts, seeds and well-prepared legumes and wholegrains.

- Fast one day each week to get a real appreciation for how little you actually need to eat (see next chapter for more on this).

- Eat at the table with friends and family, and talk instead of watching television.

- Prepare your meals ahead of time.

- Clean out the house and cupboards of all the processed foods.

- Consider eating less meat, or none at all. I stopped eating meat when I was 18, nearly 30 years ago (and my iron levels are very good, thanks).

- Improve your cooking skills.

- ENJOY YOUR FOOD!

> First of all, do not overeat. Do not be carried away by meat dishes … and never become addicted to alcohol.
>
> The oldest ever Ukrainian, Eugenia Markianovna Tebenchuk, 109 years old

What influences your food choices?

We are heavily influenced by our friends, food labels and the size of a package. The bigger something is, the more appealing it is.[5] The Framingham studies proved that happiness, smoking and obesity are all contagious. If your three best friends are obese, it is almost guaranteed that you will be overweight.

We know there is a link between sweet taste and the production of dopamine (a brain neurotransmitter that provokes feelings of pleasure) because calorie content, regardless of taste, triggers a dopamine response.[6] This shows how overeating, particularly junk foods, causes an addictive state that continues to have your brain crave overeating. This is biochemical food addiction. Junk foods laden with sugar, salt, fat and gluten trigger the same biological brain mechanisms as those in drug addicts.[7]

Sugar addicts shown their favourite foods experience a rush of dopamine to the orbital frontal cortex – the same part of the brain that responds when a cocaine addict is shown a bag of white powder. Overeat junk food and dopamine floods you with happy dopey hormones. You become completely addicted to this feeling. Junk food is as addictive as hard drugs.

Overeating

Overeating is a self-perpetuating habit, a vicious cycle that has devastatingly negative health effects. Overeating sets off a series of events that short circuit your brain appetite signals. Overeat long enough and you become totally addicted to the feelings of pleasure it gives you, and you slowly lose your ability to control any food impulses.

The hypothalamus is a cone-shaped gland, about the size of an almond, attached to the pituitary gland and lying near the brain stem. It controls hunger, as well as many other body functions. It helps the body maintain homeostasis, which is the tendency toward a stable, constant state of equilibrium. The hypothalamus dramatically alters when overeating becomes a daily habit.[8]

We know that those who eat less, who eat nutritiously and are physically active, live longer in better health, and have far lower levels of cancer, heart disease and diabetes. These most prolific killer diseases finish far too many of us before our time and are mostly preventable.

Making small changes creates new habits and this is where you will find success. The energy levels you get from eating less, the glow of your skin, the 'jump out of bed' feeling in the morning (not to mention your transformed sex life) mean that you soon get the payoff. You are healthier, stronger, leaner, more flexible, less ill, sharper in the brain and spend much less money on food and drugs.

Food is and always will be the number one critical factor in weight loss.

> True happiness is impossible without true health. True health
> is impossible without the rigid control of the palate.
>
> Mahatma Gandhi

JSB's recommendations

The following are my recommendations for losing weight and maintaining that loss over time, and for lowering your risk of all Western lifestyle diseases.

► Eat a fresh, plant-based wholefood diet.

► Eat less overall.

► Stop eating the wrong foods.

► Change your lifestyle (sleep, stress, routines).

► Low or zero alcohol intake.

► Get consistent regular daily movement.

► Regular Intelligent Fasting®.

► Stand (or move) more than you sit.

► Rebuild your gut microbiome from the inside out.

► Build your daily habits around health.

► Get your headspace/attitude/emotions in order.

► Be very clear about your SMART goals (Specific, Measurable, Achievable, Results over Time).

► Be accountable to somebody.

► Drink water between meals.

► Surround yourself with good people who support you and your goals.

Eat more plants, eat less meat

According to Dan Buettner, who has studied all of the longevity cultures around the world and calls these cultures 'The Blue Zones', all eat far less than Westerners do. They mainly eat a local, seasonal, plant-based, wholefood diet.[9] He found the following lifestyle aspects were common to all of the longest-lived cultures.

► They do not smoke.

► They move every day.

► They have daily routines and rhythms.

► They keep socially engaged and mean something to their communities.

► They eat a plant-based wholefood diet with very little or no meat.

► On average, they eat considerably less calories than Westerners do.

As a note, when you stop eating animal protein and processed foods, you may feel tired for a few days. This is normal; don't worry, as your energy will return. Most people will feel lighter and better within 24 hours. The simple solution is to not put your body through the damage in the first place, as it all leads to aging and illness.

Plant-based wholefood diets are anti-disease

We know that greatly increasing the consumption of wholesome plant foods and greatly decreasing the consumption of animal products offers profound increased longevity potential and myriad health benefits. This is mainly due to the broad symphony of life-extending phytochemical nutrients that a healthy plant-based diet contains. By taking advantage of the year-round seasonal availability of high quality plant foods, we have a unique opportunity to live both healthier and longer than ever before in human history.

Making the change

We need to change what we are eating. We have to cleanse and rebuild the body in all degenerative and acute diseases. All people with coronary heart disease, cancer and other degenerative diseases have weak or diseased livers. The only way to rebuild and strengthen the liver fully is through the diet.

Consider your liver a filter, working well with small amounts of food and liquid. However, dumping large amounts of sludge into your liver will cripple its functionality, creating blood-sugar-level problems and issues with weight. It takes three hours of very vigorous exercise to burn off the calories eaten at one small junk food session. Not eating it in the first place negates the problem entirely and saves your liver the work of damage control, also meaning it can get back to cleaning your blood, removing impurities and helping you to grow younger. And you won't need to go for that three-hour run after work or feel guilty (negative association) about your binge.

Slow and long is the only real solution for weight loss

One of the first things I learned was that I was eating too much food, which never gave my body a chance to relax and heal. I started to eat less and it has slowly become a habit. I now eat around 50% of what I used to and I have more energy, clarity, flexibility and strength. At age 46 I am as lean as I was in my 20s. It took me six years to get fully well.

Slowly change your habits. Take small, yet strong, baby steps. Give yourself a year to get well. This is the only real solution for sustainable weight loss.[10] In three months you will be feeling the difference and in 12 months, you will be reborn. I have mentored many people through this. Join our programme, thelifeplan if you would like our personal support to help you through this process.

Eat more fibre-rich plants

The crucial aspect is to eat very healthy foods since when you lose fat your body will be releasing stored toxins, such as 'persistent organic pollutants' (POPs), from the fatty tissues into the bloodstream.[11] If your diet is rich in high nutrition, plant-based wholefoods, then you are in the best position to support your immune system and remove these toxins from the body. Otherwise they may end up in your organs causing diabetes, cardiovascular disease or cancers. Exercising followed by a pig-out session never really works.

Eat more vegetables

When I changed my diet I suspected that I had to put much better nutrition into my mouth, but I did not know what that meant. I started researching and asking questions. Which foods had the crucial health-giving, body-rebuilding super nutrients? The answer, of course, was firstly, fresh vegetables and secondly, raw whole fruit. Free radical damage is one of the main causes of aging and carotenoids are the best protection we have. All the centenarian populations eat primarily vegetables and fruit, and then all of the other foods come after these two. They grow them locally and they eat them fresh and seasonally; they do not eat imported fruits and vegetables all year round.

Once scientists isolated the cluster of genes affected by caloric restriction, they began identifying the specific chemicals that activate them. What they found was that all of the important anti-aging compounds (carotenoids, vitamins, minerals and plantioxidants) that help to stimulate longevity were found predominantly in vegetables. There are many other superfoods, but vegetables are the base starting point on which all nutrition-rich, health-transforming, longevity-extending lives are built.

In the near 40-year Okinawa Centenarian Study, medical researchers said, 'Never in the history of nutrition research has the evidence been more clear and consistent; a high wholefood carbohydrate, low calorie, plant-based diet is the best for long-term health. There's no doubt about it anymore, despite what you might have read in books advocating low-carb, high animal protein diets.'

The next thing I learned was how to speed up the natural healing process in the body by fasting on freshly made vegetable juices. Miracles happen on a fast.

12
Fasting: the miracle cure

Fasting and natural diet as a therapy should be the first treatment when someone discovers that she or he has a medical problem. It should not be applied only to the most advanced cases, as is present practice. Whether the patient has a cardiac condition, hypertension, autoimmune disease, fibroids or asthma, he or she must be informed that fasting and natural, plant-based diets are a viable alternative to conventional therapy, and an effective one. The time may come when not offering this substantially more effective nutritional approach will be considered malpractice.

Dr Joel Fuhrman, MD, USA

FAST: Feel Amazing, Stimulate Transformation!

Fasting. The very word makes people go strange and make accusations that you've joined a weird cult dedicated to the worship of thin celebrities. You may very well begin reading this section of the book thinking I'm 'a bit nuts', but I'm hoping that by the time you've finished you will categorise me as a 'total health freak', which is where I belong!

Fasting is the inner doctor.

Hippocrates, father of modern medicine

They say that 'if you don't eat, you die'. The actual truth is,
'if you don't eat regularly, then you live longer'.

Jason Shon Bennett

Where to start? Just stop eating?

To be very clear, I am not recommending that you initially fast on water alone. The fasting I recommend is based on receiving a full, healthy, nutritional intake right throughout the fast. It is what I call Regular Intelligent Fasting® (RIF).

For most people, fasting as I recommend gives you more nutrition in a day than you would usually get, not less. You drink living, freshly made vegetable juice, with additional green superfoods such as spirulina, barley grass or chlorella (if desired). I have fasted this way many times over the last 30 years, and I have had the most incredible results, both in body and mind, from these experiences.

Almost everyone can benefit from RIF. It is a time for your body to clear the backlog and take a much needed break. We are living in a time where more people than ever are sick and they are getting sicker, at a younger age, all over the world. Why?

The main reason is we simply eat too much food. The secondary reason is the food we are eating is among the worst quality food ever created. The modern diet is a low fibre, sugar-rich, high meat, nutrient poor, 3500-calorie a day, gluten filled mess, prepared with processed, toxic, rancid fats. On this modern diet, your odds of dying of heart disease, cancer, diabetes, liver failure, an autoimmune disease or with mental decline in your 60s or 70s, after decades of suffering, are around 95%.

The modern diet creates nasty toxins that accumulate in our body's fat cells. Regular fasting, lifestyle changes and a healthy, balanced, plant-based wholefood diet is the best strategy to remove this waste and transform your health, vitality and longevity.

Before we begin, I'd like to make clear a few misconceptions you may have at this point. The fasting I recommend is **not**:

1. just drinking water, losing all your energy and sleeping all day

2. some kind of eating disorder to avoid food

3. some kind of 'get-stick-thin-like-a-model' programme

4. about depriving yourself of the joys in life and becoming a 'misery guts'

5. starvation (starvation is very different and damages your metabolism).

The fasting I recommend **is**:

1. Regular – you do it weekly or fortnightly or monthly.

2. Intelligent – you look after yourself while fasting, you drink vegetable juice, you get enough sleep, you manage your stress levels, you make smart lifestyle changes like not smoking or drinking (or only drinking in times of social celebration), and you see fasting as an additional support to a healthy lifestyle, not a magic bullet that recommends you eat junk foods and then fast. When you are not fasting you eat a healthy, balanced, plant-based wholefood diet.

3. Fasting – vegetable juice and water-based days.

> Fasting is the greatest remedy, the physician within.
> Instead of medication, fast for a day.
>
> Philippus Paracelsus, Greek philosopher and one of
> the three fathers of Western medicine

Fasting versus starving

Fasting is taking in water or liquid-based sustenance over a period of time. Fasting is allowing your body to digest and remove the stored fuel it is carrying as fat. Each half kilogram of extra fat you carry is stored fuel and is equivalent to 3500 calories or two days' food supply. Most people have plenty of stored fuel all over their bodies. Just look down at your belly, or your thighs, or your bum, or feel your neck.

RIF is not malnourishment or starvation. Even if you do fast for a day on water alone, most people have plenty of calories stored to carry them through those 24 hours and probably for much longer. Water-only fasting is discussed later in this book. Long-term starvation weakens the body, but RIF strengthens the body. Fasting may not be appropriate for those people (actually very few in Western society) who are underweight with a very low BMI and low energy, until weight is gained. (See my recommendations about who should or should not fast later in this chapter.)

Starvation is very different to fasting. Starvation is when your body has no fuel, no fat or nutrient reserves, and then you stop eating. I do not recommend starvation.

Regular Intelligent Fasting®

RIF is what I suggest you do. For the rest of your life, regularly fast intelligently, not stupidly and not when it is inappropriate. RIF is what many of the great leaders, teachers, philosophies and religions have taught for over 2000 years, in an effort to achieve exceptional health.

Fasting is the best medicine, the original cure. This is why you naturally lose your appetite when you are sick. Fasting is simply the oldest, most powerful, historically proven, immediate and effective, natural rejuvenation process available.

The organs in the human body are designed to work for 120 years, but they are vastly overworked during our lives, mainly due to overeating. Fasting exerts a normalising effect on all physiological functions, be they mental, glandular, hormonal, biochemical or mineral. Fasting is energising, invigorating and revitalising and is one of the safest healing methods known to man or medical science. Fasting is the best way to grow younger, cleanse internally and to give your body a well deserved holiday. RIF is ideal for controlling and managing weight because it changes the chemistry in your body and improves your metabolism.

A healthy person can survive without food for 50–75 days.

A. J. Carlson, Professor of Physiology, University of Chicago, USA

Why fast?

When you break a leg, what do you do with it? You rest it so it can heal. When you are exhausted, what do you do? You rest so you can recover. When your digestive and bowel system is clogged, what do you do? You fast, so your engine room, your digestive system and your entire body can rest, recover, rebuild, reboot, refresh, rejuvenate and revitalise. You feel reborn.

Fasting is to recovery what sleep is to recuperation. For me, discovering fasting has been one of the key health-changing moments in my sickness to health journey. Slowly starting to fast, gently at first, and then more rigorously over time, will for most people completely transform their health.

Babies and animals naturally fast when unwell

Fasting is second nature to babies and animals. Human babies, when sick, will immediately fast. Animals automatically avoid food and fast to ease pain, discomfort or disease. When ill, animals will instinctively find a source of clean water, then rest by it and fast. Dogs have been known to fast up to 60 days. When we get sick, we lose our appetite. This is your body begging you to fast so it can concentrate on fixing the problem.

The real problem is not fasting. The real problem is that we keep eating.

Fasting is in our blood

Our bodies are actually designed to go for days without eating. From an evolutionary standpoint, the human body is 99.98% identical to what it was 10,000 generations ago. We did not evolve with constant access to food because the food supply was sporadic. When food was plentiful, we ate more than we required and stored the excess as fat. When times were scarce, we would fast and survive on our fat stores. Our bodies adapted to this over time and the process kept our bodies in a constant state of preparedness. During the Paleolithic period, humans did not eat nearly as regularly as we do now, and on average about one day per week they would go without any food at all.

You can live for months without solid food, for 70 days without any food, or you can kill yourself in just a few days by overeating.

An historical overview

Throughout our long and varied medicinal history, fasting has been regarded as one of the most dependable, curative and rejuvenative measures available. Galen prescribed it. Paracelsus called fasting 'the greatest remedy, the physician within.' The father of medicine, Hippocrates, found that fasting, 'helped the body heal itself', and wrote a great deal about its incredible medicinal potential. Plato said, 'I fast to attain greater mental and physical efficiency.' Fasting has been practiced by many great philosophers and thinkers such as Socrates, Mahatma Gandhi, Aristotle, Jesus Christ and Dr Martin Luther King.

Most world religions have recommended fasting as a way to cure illness, improve physical health and attain spiritual clarity. Many cultures include fasting as part of their discipline because of its freeing effect on the mind as well as the role it plays in self-discipline. The Bible and the Koran make frequent recommendations about the benefits of regular fasting. Buddhism,

Hinduism, Christianity, Judaism, Islam, the ancient Essene, Chinese medicine and Ayurveda teachings all recommend fasting for physical and mental health.

When ancient people had to go without food, they carried on because this was life as usual. Throughout human evolution there have always been periods of famine and when there is famine you have two choices: fast or die. We are built to fast while sick or unwell. Without fasting we would not be here, as our ancestors would have died. We are the genetic children of fasting generations throughout history. There has always been a safe and healthy place for fasting throughout our evolution. The only generations not to fast regularly have been those born after the year 1900.

In 1978, Edmond Bordeaux Szekely published his religious book, *The Essene Science of Fasting*. In his book, he gave a thorough overview of fasting. He said, 'Fasting is the most ancient therapy of humanity. Even our forefathers observed that after some days of fasting, a recrudescence of vitality and vigor shows itself in the organism. Nature turns it to account for the purpose of accelerating the functions and by the vital machine's slackened activity resulting from the fast to cast off the impurities of the organism by every channel ... I do not know of any therapeutic method which can be as effective as the fast. It is sad but none the less true, that generally we eat very much more than is necessary for the organism as regards both quantity and quality. Fasting is a radical cure which counterbalances the evil effects of overeating and unwise choice of food.'

The father of American naturopathy, Dr Benedict Lust (1872–1945), was a strong advocate of fasting. The famous and well-respected Dr Bernard Jensen (1908–2001) recommended fasting at his Hidden Valley Health Ranch in the hills outside Escondido, California. Presently, the International Association of Hygienic Physicians (IAHP) specialises in therapeutic fasting. My team and I also offer fasting retreats where we take you through a fast and teach you how in a way you can do at home yourself for the rest of your life. We also give RIF support every week as part of our health mentoring programme, thelifeplan.

We're not good at responding to too many calories but we're very good at responding to fasting. Fasting, in itself, is not an unhealthy process. During fasting, almost every system in the body is 'turned down', the body changes how it uses fuel, certain hormone levels fall, growth stops. By the end of three weeks of fasting, you are a completely different metabolic creature. It affects many, many processes but in a somewhat predictable way that takes you towards disease prevention.

Dr Marc Hellerstein, Professor of Endocrinology, Metabolism and Nutrition, University of California

Be well before you fast, do not fast to be well

You must be well before you attempt to fast. I recommend you eat a plant-based wholefood diet, improve your bowel motions, get plenty of sleep, adjust your lifestyle such that you have a handle on your stress exposure, and give up smoking and drinking (drinking is there for rare and celebratory social occasions not as a daily ritual) before fasting.

Doing this before you start fasting will make your fasting experience very different because your bowel will be healthier. Currently, I can fast for a day easily if I feel like it. This is because I have the other areas of my health taken care of.

Fasting must be adapted to the individual. Some people take years before they are well enough to fast easily and regularly. Other people can water-fast immediately for a day and then continue this practice for the rest of their lives.

Be gentle with yourself. There is plenty of time. I highly recommend getting yourself relatively healthy before you begin the practice of Regular Intelligent Fasting®.

13
Why fast?

The question should really be 'Why not fast?', given the historically proven unique health benefits that are available only through fasting.

Jason Shon Bennett

What is a fast?

Technically, fasting is any condition in which the body is encouraged to initiate the process of autolysis, or self digestion. A fast usually means drinking only liquid without eating any food at all for a period of time. Fasting can be done whenever you like. I recommend irregular RIF for one full day each week. Vary the day so the body does not adjust and get used to it. I also recommend fasting for one full week or more as suits you (7–14 days), once every season.

Fasting is done for therapeutic reasons: to cure illness, rebalance the body, prevent disease, kickstart a new habit, or to lose excessive weight. Fasting on vegetable juices or only one food (apple juice, for example) is called 'juice fasting' or a 'monodiet'. How well the fast is done, and how well you eat after the fast, determines how good the results. Fasting starts around 12 hours after a meal. At this stage you have used up the available glucose in your blood and the body starts converting glycogen stored in the liver and muscle cells into glucose for energy.

> We must restore fasting to the place it occupied in an ancient
> hierarchy of values 'above medicine'. We must rediscover it
> and restore it to honour because it is a necessity.
>
> The Buchinger Clinics, Germany

Fasting can create miracles

I have fasted hundreds of times over 25 years, from simple one-day fasts to a life-changing mega-31-day fast. I have experienced so many benefits including increased energy levels, improved digestion, loss of bloating, younger skin, removal of impacted bowel waste, weight loss, asthma symptoms disappearing, creative songwriting episodes and clarity of thought. Fasting is superb for getting your health back. Almost everyone I know at some stage has asked me about the experience and benefits of fasting. Questions I'm consistently asked include, 'What did you eat on your last fast?', 'How long do you think I should fast for?', 'What do I expect on a fast?' and 'How do I fast safely and intelligently?'

Most people are really interested in the benefits that fasting offers but do not know where to start. Currently, many naturopathic colleges are not teaching their students about fasting so the knowledge is being lost. The media, and some nutritional experts, say fasting is dangerous and advise you never to do it. They think it is something negative because they are uninformed about fasting. Fasting is in our genes and is the most natural thing for human beings this side of eating.

> Fasting, woohoo! I've just done three days of juice fasting, the
> longest I've managed so far. I feel wonderful, cleaner in the body
> and the mind. It was only going to be one day but I was feeling
> good so I thought I'd see how far I could go, and I think the body
> needed a good rest. Actually, that's been a key change in my
> thinking, I now look at fasting as resting and being 'kind to my
> digestive system' rather than starving myself, so that's a big
> change for me! So weird, I thought I'd feel moody and horrible
> but it's the complete reverse, I'm so glad I tried it.
>
> Antoinette, on thelifeplan, 2012

The benefits of fasting

The Top 10 benefits

1. Provides a much-needed rest for internal organs.
2. Accelerates the elimination of diseased, decaying, dying or dead cells.
3. Rebuilds your intestinal bowel health.
4. Breaks the gluten, fat, sugar and salt (GFSS) food addictions.
5. Restores normal glandular, hormonal and metabolic rates.
6. Completely transforms the skin.
7. Reduces pain and inflammation in the body.
8. Improves cellular oxygenation and nutritional uptake.
9. Alkalises and relaxes the nervous system.
10. Lowers serum fats (which restores vitality to the organs).

Fasting improves resistance to illness, leaving you stronger, healthier and younger. Dr Ragnar Berg, Nobel Prize winner, was perhaps the world's greatest food scientist and most highly regarded authority on nutrition and biochemistry. He fasted many times and had supervised many fasts. He said, 'During fasting the body burns up and excretes huge amounts of accumulated wastes. We can help this cleansing process by drinking alkaline juices instead of water while fasting. I have supervised many fasts and made extensive tests of fasting patients, and I am convinced that drinking alkaline-forming fruit and vegetable juices instead of water, during fasting, will increase the healing effect of fasting. Elimination of uric acid and other inorganic acids will be accelerated. And sugars in juices will strengthen the heart ... Juice fasting is the best form of fasting.'

When fasting, the body switches on the 'inner nutrition' and starts burning rubbish as fuel. This fuel is contained in every cell and every organ, in the form of glycogen in the liver, protein in the blood/lymph system, stored fat (even in thin people), and assorted food elements in the bone marrow and glands. The miracle is that the body will first burn those cells that are damaged, diseased, dying or dead, which I like to call the 4Ds. The body will feed on and remove fat deposits containing pesticides, medicines, drugs, additives, toxins, tumours, dead tissues, uric acid and useless accumulations. The essential organs like the brain and nervous system are not eaten (a good thing!).

Fasting cuts the body some slack

Fasting is primarily effective because it gives the body a genuine chance to rest, recover, rebuild and refresh. Specifically, the digestive organs (stomach, liver, kidneys, intestines and bowels) are given a rare break from the continual digestion of food. Up to 60% of the energy you have at any one time can be spent on digestion, so this saved energy can be used for healing, cell growth, regeneration, cleansing and the rebuilding of your immune system. During fasting, serum magnesium (very beneficial) is increased through the body. Also important is that without food any inflammation from junk foods is avoided. Fasting can be helpful whether someone is overweight or within their appropriate weight range. Fasting one day each week provides the same advantages as long-term calorie restriction and makes the body more sensitive to insulin, which helps maintain normal blood-sugar levels.

Fasting helps boost almost all body functions

Studies have demonstrated the tremendous beneficial effects of fasting on the various human body functions, particularly on the gastrointestinal (digestive) and cardiovascular (heart) systems. Fasting does not affect the working of the brain because mental work does not require extra energy. Your brain consumes equal amounts of glucose and oxygen whether you are awake, asleep, eating or fasting.

Fasting adjusts your genes for the better. For example, a 'transcription factor' protein called Foxa2 activates and stimulates a different genetic expression. Foxa2 influences fat burning, sleep, intake of food and sexual behavior. When fasting there is a lack of insulin and Foxa2 becomes active, making you more alert and physically active.[1] This is clever design because when there was no food, the body needed you to go out looking for food! Fasting makes you more active so you can get up, get out and walk, run and climb to secure more food – so you survive!

As we discovered earlier, the Ikarian people in Greece regularly fast. It serves them well as they have the best longevity rates and the lowest rates of disease anywhere in Europe. Nearly 30% of all Ikarians live into their 90s. They have 50% lower rates of heart disease and 20% the cancer rates of those in the West. They have near-zero cases of dementia. Ikarians not only live a long time, but they also live well. They party hard, have healthy sexual relationships into their 90s, walk everywhere, are very active, sleep when they feel tired, fast regularly, have low levels of stress and eat significantly less than most Europeans.[2]

Strangely I am feeling fine. I realize we don't need to eat
every day. And we certainly don't need three meals a day.
I feel so well that I'm bored.

Mia Farrow, actress, after ten days' fasting

Fasting and the removal of body waste

Fasting automatically engages our rejuvenation systems to perform a variety of truly incredible tasks. Fasting speeds up the elimination of toxic wastes and dead cells, accelerates new cell and tissue generation, and enhances cell oxygenation. Fasting cleanses the bowel and restores vitality to organs and nervous systems. Fasting specifically prevents more toxic substances from entering the body. It allows for the expulsion of stored toxins, for example, the uric acid sticking around the joints diagnosed as gout arthritis, and heavy metals stored in the fat cells. Fasting restores and normalises glandular, metabolic and nervous system functions.

Due to processed foods in our diets, environmental pollutants and stress, most of us suffer from toxic deposits throughout the body. With fasting speeding up the elimination of these toxins, remarkable and sometimes incredible changes can occur. Even if you are relatively healthy, a fast is a wonderful preventative measure against aging and possible future disease. Some medical experts say that fasting helps to 'reset' the cells of the body to a neutral state, thus allowing the body's systems to function and perform more efficiently. The body holds on to important minerals and vitamins when throwing out toxins and old tissues. When the toxic load of the body is lessened, the efficiency of each cell is enhanced.

Fasting is a refuse disposal, a burning of rubbish.

Dr Otto Buchinger Senior, one of the world's greatest fasting authorities, Germany

How does fasting work?

Fasting is a very complicated physiological process and this chapter is not a thorough or completely detailed scientific explanation of it. For that you would need a 1000-page medical book on fasting! However, the following is a very basic overview of what happens when you fast.

Day 1

After your cells have used up all the available fuel in the bloodstream, your body turns to your liver and your muscles, where sugar is stored as glycogen. You start lipolysis, which is the body burning through your glycogen reserves to make glucose. This usually takes 16–24 hours.

Day 2

When your body has no more glycogen to burn, it turns to autolysis (self digestion), which is when the body starts eating old and diseased, dying, decaying or dead cells, for energy. Gluconeogenesis (GNG) also starts, which is when the body converts and recycles the old proteins to glycogen, for energy. Gluconeogenesis is a natural liver process in humans and animals and can happen during fasting or intense exercise.

Day 3

Ketogenesis (sometimes called ketosis) kicks in, which is when the liver breaks down body fat stores into ketones, to be used by the brain, red blood cells, heart and muscles. This helps preserve the body's protein stores and happens when there are no carbohydrates supplied through diet. As fat is increasingly burned as fuel, fat-stored toxins are released into the bloodstream to be metabolised by the liver and kidneys, and to be processed as waste. Ketones are very acidic, but during intelligent fasting the blood is far more balanced and alkaline. While fasting the blood can buffer this acidity to keep the blood pH normal and healthy. Too many accumulated ketones in the blood and you have ketogenesis.

Ketogenesis is a very natural metabolic adaptation process, otherwise known as 'muscle sparing'. You lose less than 200 grams of muscle per day once full ketogenesis is reached (usually by the third day of water fasting), but this varies enormously depending on how much body fat you are carrying. If you are generally healthy this small muscle loss is negligible. The natural sugars in juice fasting prevent ketogenesis from occurring.

Day 4 onwards

Your stomach shrinks and your appetite drops. This is where juice fasting becomes fun as a glass of juice is as filling as a big dinner. You also start to experience increased energy levels and a heightened sense of awareness and clarity of mind.

14

My experience of fasting

Fasting simply changes everything ...

Jason Shon Bennett

My first experience

The very first time I fasted I was, as the saying goes, as sick as a dog. I fasted for seven days and all I could do was lie around. I was totally unaware of my diet leading up to this first fast, so I literally went from takeaway burgers, chips, soft drinks and junk foods to fresh fruit juices and vegetable juices overnight. Was I ill! My nose ran, my skin broke out, I vomited a great deal and my bum did not stop. I had so much stuff to come out, and my body had never been given a break before. I don't know how I mustered up the energy, but my first child, Trey, was conceived during that fast (woohoo!). I completely forgot about contraception because my head was such a mess. Trey was the best thing to come out of that first fast, now that I come to think of it ... totally changed my life that boy did. He is still a huge inspiration to me.

However, in hindsight, it would have been much better to get myself relatively healthy and fit before that fast, which is why I am telling you this story.

Fasting, for me, has been the single most revelatory and powerful experience I have ever had, or learnt about, in almost 30 years of studying and researching health. It helped cure my asthma, my

digestive system, my skin and my back; improved my flexibility and
peace of mind; and broke my food addictions and weight problems.

Jason Shon Bennett

My longest fast

Over the last 25 years I have fasted regularly for periods from 1 to 33 days. I
have varied the mixture of water, herbal teas, vegetable juices, green superfood
powders and occasionally some fresh fruit juices/vegetable protein powders/
nuts and seeds, depending on circumstance and ingredients at hand. The
longest fast I did in my 20s was 31 days.

The longest fast I have done so far was 31 days. This fast was interesting
for a number of reasons. Firstly, for the fact that all I did was juice fruits in
the mornings and vegetables in the afternoons. No spirulina, no superfoods,
no fibre added and no wholefood liquid supplements. Nothing else but
fresh fruit juices or fresh vegetable juices. I have never fasted like that since.
Secondly, I worked at my job in a health store right through the fast. I was
carrying 25 kg bags of oats, making muesli in a concrete mixer (probably
would not get away with that nowadays) and riding my bike to work each
day. Thirdly, I had incredible creative bursts on this fast. I wrote songs, my
brain was working overtime and I had many lyrics and melodies pouring out
of me, especially during the last few days, when I penned one of the best
songs I have ever written called 'True Freedom'.

I was also doing enemas, which involves a special kit with a long tube that
is inserted into the anus and is connected to a water bag. You fill your bowels
with liquid, lie down and massage your tummy for a while and then go to
the toilet, where it all (and much more) comes out. Today you can now get
this procedure, known as colonic irrigation, done commercially. I thoroughly
recommend it to anyone serious about bowel health.

However, the most interesting thing about this mega 31-day fast was
what came out of my bowels on the morning of day 31. I woke up and felt
the urge to go number twos. Remember, this is after 31 days of nothing
but juiced fruit or vegetable. As I sat on the toilet and strained, the longest,
blackest, driest poo I have ever done came out. I could not believe it! It must
have taken 30 minutes to get that three-foot-long sucker out of me! It was all
I could do to look down between my legs, mouth agape, thinking, 'Where the
hell has this come from?' The faeces was dry like sandpaper, completely black
and had no smell that I can recall. It had been wrapped around my bowels,

slowing me down and suffocating my ability to get enough good nutrition from my food, regardless of the quality. My asthma disappeared soon after. In hindsight, I wish I had vac-packed it so I could show people what can get lodged in the intestines. However, I think I was in shock and I flushed that momentous movement away.

What was that black thing? What exactly was it that takes 31 days of fresh juice fasting, daily stomach massages and enemas to get out? I knew that many people had between one and seven kgs of undigested faecal matter stuck in their colon, but this was ridiculous. It was the all-time whopper of poos. It looked like a big, black snake that had been beaten up by Muhammad Ali, put through a washing machine, and then dehydrated! I could not believe that something like that had been sitting inside me.

It was at this moment that I truly understood how far out of balance our bowels can become. As red meat and hard yellow cheese both constipate me (and most people), I suspect it was some disgusting toxic glue-based mixture of meat, cheese and gluten I ate as a kid that had stuck to the sides of my bowels. I have never, ever, looked at my bowels the same way again.

Connecting what I had been eating all my life to my body-wide sickness, my low immunity, my many and varied health problems and my constipation was a light bulb moment. I realised how important it was to look after my bowels and digestive system. They are our engine room, the key part of the body that builds everything else.

My health has never been the same since that fast. Not only did my skin change, my bowels started changing, so much so that I now go three times a day easily and without straining (I used to go once, with straining), my asthma went away, my breathing and my bloating changed, but most important of all: my relationship with food changed, forever.

My water fasting

The longest water fast I have done is six days. It was fascinating as I functioned completely normally. Nobody around me knew (unless I told them), and the only thing I did differently was not exercising as rigorously. My bowels were so clean afterwards that in the following days whenever I ate I would eliminate within 30 minutes. Just like a baby.

Water fasting is like an internal shower, cleaning the body from within. I water fast for a few days to start all my fasts now, but I do not recommend water fasting until you are highly experienced at juice fasting.

Fourteen days of water-fasting, winter 2013

In 2013, I did a two-week fast during winter that was just water, the occasional fresh vegetable juice, ginger water (freshly grated ginger simmered in hot water), pure herbal teas, some spirulina and chlorella powder, and occasionally a little soaked linseed to keep the bowels moving. I walked almost every day right through this fast, often a distance of 11 kilometres, which included ascending the side of one of Auckland's favourite volcano sites, Cornwall Park. On day 13, I walked through the bush to the top of Cornwall Park with a two kg weight on each leg. On day 14 I woke at 5 a.m., swam one hundred lengths of the local pool (two kilometres in 50 minutes), then walked in the Albany bush for an hour. On day 15 I woke at 5 a.m., did my full yoga workout and, for the first time in two-and-a-half years, I managed to touch both arms behind my back again (a classic yoga pose). In January 2011 I had injured my shoulder badly and had never gotten close to this level of flexibility. I thought I might never get it back, but after two weeks on mainly water it was healed. This was unbelievable given I had gone to many back specialists over the preceding two years with no results.

Fasting is a rebirth and a cleanse

Many of the toxic chemicals we ingest are fat soluble (marijuana, for example), and store in our fatty tissue such as the brain and endocrine glands. This debris can accumulate in the body for years to our detriment, but can be released during fasting. Fasting is great if you use it to kick off a new start or an improvement to your daily habits. If you do it once a year and go back to pigging out and eating rubbish, then you are wasting your time and doing more harm than good. The human body works on long-term consistency. Small changes that last are much better for you than fasting once and then troffing on anti-nutrient, junk food pig-outs.

I am not a fan of 'detoxing' as a separate experience. I am a fan of the regular daily and weekly discipline of treating yourself well. Hence, what I promote and recommend is Regular Intelligent Fasting®. Eating well, getting well and staying well is what I recommend. RIF is a key part of staying well – for the rest of your life.

Hence, what I promote and recommend is Regular Intelligent Fasting®. RIF is a key part of staying well – for the rest of your life. As I write this, in November 2013, I am on day 33 of a fast (my longest fast ever!). I feel amazing, my skin is glowing and I am walking so quickly (while still carrying weights) that Tracey cannot keep up!

15
Fasting, the liver, and your skin

Liver health

I recommend fasting one day each week to support long-term health. The problem with doing a detox to clean the liver is that people do it, get cleaned up and then go back to their bad habits. Every time I fast, I go back to food with a fresh perspective and appreciation of how to look after myself better. It is always a reminder of how little food I actually require to be vital and healthy. Your vitality, health and longevity are closely linked to the health of your liver.

What does the liver do?

The liver completely regenerates every 10 to 20 months, so you can clean and rebuild it with good food, exercise, water and fasting. The liver is the largest organ in the body, positioned under the lower right ribcage. It is the major blood reservoir, filtering more than 1.4 litres of blood per minute. Every single drop of blood passes through the liver for inspection. This means all the good and essential nutrients as well as the impurities and toxins we have ingested end up there. The liver is one of the cornerstones to a person's physical and mental vitality.

The liver manufactures and stores nutrients, regulates metabolism and processes protein for new cells, hormones and enzymes. It changes the carbohydrate foods we eat into glucose and glycogen for energy. It converts fat into insulating and protective tissue, and runs the detoxification of poisons and disposal of wastes. It removes bacteria, toxic chemicals, drugs, hormones and various other unwanted substances from the body via the bowels, lungs, kidneys or skin, and converts fat soluble chemicals into water soluble chemicals to be removed via bile or the urine. Like any filter, the liver can become overworked and blocked with impurities. If you do not jump out of bed in the morning feeling relatively awake and clear headed, then your liver is struggling. I call this having a 'sugar liver' from too much alcohol, processed food, animal products or refined sugar,and not enough water and fibre rich leafy green vegetables.

> The food we eat should be our medicine. Our medicine for
> our body should be our food. But to eat when you are sick
> is to feed your sickness.
>
> Hippocrates, MD, 460–377 BC

The biggest cause of death on earth is heart disease

Heart disease death is mostly preventable and heart disease is strongly linked to fatty liver disease. Half of all Westerners over the age of 50 have a sick, fatty, unwell liver. Fatty liver disease is all about diet and alcohol. Heart disease is all about diet and alcohol, so it stands to reason that they are linked. Dr Rajiv Chhabra, a gastroenterologist at Saint Luke's Health System's Liver Disease Management Center, recommends that 'Patients with coronary artery disease should be screened for liver disease, and likewise [patients with non-alcoholic fatty liver disease] should be evaluated for coronary artery disease.'[1]

In 2013, Dr Chhabra and Dr John Helzberg found a strong link between non-alcoholic fatty liver disease and high risk for heart disease in their research. On scanning and testing over 400 patients, they saw that those with non-alcoholic fatty liver disease were far more likely to have coronary artery disease.[1] Here is the real kicker, though: the influence of non-alcoholic fatty liver disease on heart disease risk was **stronger** than all the other classic markers for heart disease such as smoking, high blood pressure, diabetes, high cholesterol, metabolic syndrome or 'being male'.

So what changes, reverses and, in many cases, cures, fatty liver disease? Regular fasting, lifestyle changes and a plant-based wholefood diet.

If current trends continue the prevalence of non-alcoholic fatty liver disease is expected to increase to 40% of the population by 2020.

Dr John Helzberg, Saint Luke's Health System, New York

Alcohol and weight

A massive international study published in 2013[2] confirmed that alcohol and excessive weight directly lead to fatal liver diseases and liver cancer. In this study, 'low alcohol intake' was classed as two standard drinks per day and a high intake as over two drinks daily. Major findings in the study included the following.

▶ Being overweight and drinking alcohol triples the risk of fatal liver disease in women compared to slim non-drinkers.

▶ Liver disease is now the fifth-biggest killer in the alcohol-drenched UK.

▶ There was a tenfold increase in death from cirrhosis among middle-aged women in England from 1970–2000.

▶ Liver disease death has risen by 20% over the past decade.

▶ There are often no warning signs of liver disease until it is too late to treat.

▶ Those with alcoholic cirrhosis or fatty liver disease, who are overweight or obese or who have type II diabetes, are all far more likely to develop the most common liver cancer, hepatocellular carcinoma or HCC.

▶ In Europe, one in seven adults drink more than the advised limit.

The combination of a woman's drinking habits and weight has an important effect on liver health and life expectancy. Women with high alcohol intake have a greater risk of developing chronic liver disease compared to a woman who doesn't drink very much. Women are twice as sensitive as men to alcohol related liver damage and developing a more severe form of the disease at lower doses with shorter durations of alcohol consumption. Fatty liver and alcohol have long been known as risk factors for liver cancer.

Daniele Prati, European Association for the Study of the Liver (EASL)

> In my opinion, regular fasts are far more conductive to
> rejuvenation than monkey- or goat-gland transplantations,
> hormone injections, facelifts, massive vitamin intakes, or
> any other extreme or expensive measures used 'to turn
> back the clock'.
>
> Dr Alan Cott, MD, *Fasting – the Ultimate Diet*

Fasting and your liver

Many different and combined factors determine whether the liver performs its critical functions well. Too much pressure on the liver from overeating, too much rich, acidic or poor quality food, or environmental pollution and emotional stress, can all cause liver overload. This leads to a decreased ability to clear toxins and hormones and to manufacture bile. The overloaded liver then allows toxic waste material to pass into the blood and the body.

Fasting gives the liver a break and allows it to get some internal house-cleaning done. Instead of survival it turns its attention to burning up the long-term stored rubbish. The enzymes in our blood usually focus on digestion. When we fast, these enzymes move from the gut into the bloodstream, where they immediately begin purifying internal systems. They eat and break down old, damaged cells and eliminate them. Fasting gives the liver a breather from its usual 24/7 cleaning processes.

The cellular regeneration process

You are only as old or as young as your cellular structure. Life is only as vital as its weakest parts, so your health depends on your smallest vital links: your cells. Aging begins when your normal process of cell regeneration and rebuilding slows down. This is caused by the accumulation of waste products in the intestines and, therefore, the tissues. This 'glug' limits the ability of the cells to receive nutrition and nourishment. Every cell in your body needs a consistent supply of nutrition because they are unique entities with their own metabolisms and life cycles. When this process is interrupted, incapacitated or regularly disturbed, your body starts to grow old. Generally, this happens from simply eating too much food.

Due to the effects of fasting, a fast can help you heal with greater
speed; cleanse your liver, kidneys, and colon; purify your blood;

> help you lose excess weight and water; flush out toxins;
> clear the eyes and tongue; and cleanse the breath.
>
> Dr James F. Balch, MD, *Prescription for Nutritional Healing*

Fasting causes cellular regeneration

The ultimate state of youthful health and energy is achieved when there is a perfect balance in this cellular regeneration process. If your cells are breaking down and dying at a faster pace than new cells are being created, then rapid aging appears. Effective, regular and quick removal of the dead cells stimulates the growth and development of new cells.

Every one of your ten trillion body cells is at a different stage: 50% are at their peak, they are vital, effective, working and rebuilding the body; 25% are in growth and development; and 25% are in the stage of dying, decay, disease, death and removal.

While fasting, serum fats in the blood decrease, which thins the blood. Thinner blood increases oxygenation of tissues and enhances the delivery of white blood cells throughout the body. When you fast, you force the body to look elsewhere than the gut for energy. Body cells turn to damaged or older proteins for energy. Amino acids from proteins are not wasted when fasting, but are changed from one state to another. New cells are rebuilt from old, decomposed cells. The body uses the free time and energy to recognise old non-essential tissues and dissolve them, while recycling their important nutrients for new cell production. This means that when you eat again the cell will be able to use the new food components to replace the older ones it consumed. The building of new cells is vastly stimulated and increased when fasting. This means you grow more new, fresh young cells to replace old, dying cells. You are, literally, growing younger.

> I must say in all seriousness that fasting, when combined with a properly selected diet, is the nearest approach to a 'cure-all' that is possible to conceive – profoundly simple and simply profound!
>
> Dr John Tilden, MD, USA

Fasting: the single most powerful and successful way to grow younger

Fasting initiates cellulite removal. Excess saturated fat, margarine, hydrogenated, trans-fat oils or fat-based toxins are all dumped in the fat cells to keep them away from the vital organs. They make your fat cells stagnate.

These oil variations are totally unnecessary, nutritionally useless and what is more, damage and age us. They can show up on our body as cellulite. They require a large supply of good fats/oils to neutralise them.

Fasting with a mixture of soaked nuts and/or seeds means the body can focus on neutralising and removing these cellulite deposits in the most efficient way possible. Fasting has a rejuvenating effect on all the vital internal organs, including the functions of the all-important endocrine glands, which are responsible for how young or old you feel and look. During fasting the endocrine glands release toxic chemicals stored in fatty tissue for removal, making you look and feel younger.

Fasting and your skin

The most amazing thing you notice while fasting is the improvement in the quality of your skin. According to Dr Joel Fuhrman MD, clinical observations show psoriasis and psoriatic arthritis respond very favourably to fasting. In one medical study, 80% of patients noted improvement in their psoriasis after a seven- to ten-day fast.

The more I have fasted on freshly made vegetable juice, the nut and/or seed mixture, green superfoods, green tea, herb teas and lots of water, the younger I have looked. It is an absolute miracle cure for aging, wrinkles, lines, a dud liver, old-looking skin and a run-down face. My skin has never been better or more youthful than when I have been fasting. Wrinkles and lines on my face have disappeared. The only time in my adult life that I have been wrinkle free and line free on my face, even after developing wrinkles, has been while fasting. Fasting makes your liver happy and when your liver is happy, your skin is happy.

When fasting, your cells go into a kind of hibernation. Their aging process slows down dramatically, meaning your aging process slows down. This is a cooling, slowing effect, like keeping food in the fridge. You get increased healthy SIRT1 (a sirtuin enzyme) levels.[3] Fasting causes SIRT1 to stop the body generating fats and cholesterol.[4] Not bad, aye?

16

Fasting and weight loss

The relationship we have with food is so basic and so primal that most of the time we do not question it. We have been raised by generations who felt they did not ever quite have enough food due to wars, famines or economic downturns. We used to 'have to' fast but now, we have to think and turn our brains on to escape the constant overwhelming, overeating culture that is all around us and is all pervasive.

Jason Shon Bennett

Fasting, metabolism and weight loss

Human growth hormone (HGH) is the most important fat hormone in your body. It decreases body fat, reduces insulin levels, increases insulin sensitivity, and boosts muscle tissue. When fasting the production of this hormone is stimulated, resulting in higher amounts of fat being burned. HGH levels increase by 10 to 20 times when you are fasting.[1]

Benjamin Horne, of the Intermountain Heart Institute in Murray, Utah, found that one full day water fast, performed monthly, raises levels of human growth hormone (HGH). The higher level of HGH means more fat-burning enzymes are created. Adipose tissue 'hormone-sensitive lipase' (HSL) encourages fat cells to release fat for your muscles to use as energy. Muscle tissue lipoprotein lipase (LPL) helps your muscles uptake the fat to burn as fuel.

Fasting increases the release of both adipose and muscle tissue and influences other hormones to create a fantastic fat-burning environment. In my own case studies and in varied medically supervised research, fasting one day per week has been shown to be a novel and effective strategy for weight loss, hypertension and cardiovascular protection.[2] It is ideal for your heart and balancing your weight. Eating less and/or fasting regularly increases fat burning and whole-body fat oxidation rates.[3]

Molecules, cells and your size

In one fasting study, of 377 metabolites, hormones, enzymes and other signalling molecules analysed, 44% positively changed after fasting for 36 hours.[4] This is almost half of all these health markers changing for the better, after fasting for a day and two nights. This length of time is what I recommend clients begin with in RIF.

In the fasting study, the levels of the satiety hormone, leptin, decreased in the blood. The highest levels of blood leptin are found in obese people. When you fast regularly, this drops and resets your genuine appetite back to a healthy, natural level. Fasting benefits the entire body.

> Conventional nutrition experts would suggest those fasting would experience a slowed metabolism, cannibalized lean body mass, and increased body fat. But would that make evolutionary sense? Why would our bodies develop a response to scarcity that promoted physical infirmity, weakness, and decreased mobility? If we were without food, wouldn't it make sense for our bodies to conserve strength and burn fat for energy, rather than reduce it and burn muscle? In a tight spot like possible starvation, we needed that strength more than ever.
>
> Mark Sisson, *The Primal Blueprint*

Fasting and your metabolism

Many studies have now confirmed that for most people, a three-day fast does not significantly alter the metabolism, and in some cases it improves it.[5] Fasting for one to three days can boost your metabolism and adrenaline levels, burning more calories. The more calories you burn, the faster you lose weight. Fasting has a beneficial effect on weight loss and metabolism in healthy and overweight people.[6] The human body needs the same amount of energy for its daily operations, regardless of whether you are fasting or not –just as a car needs the same amount of fuel regardless of how much you have in the tank. You burn around 100 less calories per day when fasting, which makes almost no difference to your metabolism. There is a slight reduction in core body temperature, but that is about it. Following a drop in blood sugar level and using the reserves of glucose found in liver glycogen, the basal metabolic rate (BMR) is mildly reduced in order to conserve as much energy within the body as can be provided.

Juice fasting and weight loss

Vegetable juice fasting is the oldest, quickest and safest biochemical method of shedding unwanted weight and increasing your physical health. Regular juice fasting helps you to stay slim, healthy and vital, and is a huge help in the breaking of food addictions. Just one glass of vegetable juice a day helps with weight loss.[7] Drinking a glass of freshly squeezed juice every morning lowers the risk of obesity.[8] The best juices for weight loss are grapefruit or celery juices as they are lower in calories than other fruit juices and contain higher levels of soluble fibre.

Grapefruit

Grapefruit burns body fat more effectively than any other food on earth. Freshly made grapefruit juice is the only liquid in the plant kingdom that will break down the same amount of fat. Grapefruit is fairly low in calories (74 calories per cup). It is the only food that contains the antioxident naringenin, the ultimate fat burner. This bitter pigment triggers the liver to trigger your genes to break down stored fat in the human body. Naringenin targets a group of nuclear receptor proteins called peroxisome proliferator-activated receptors (PPARs). PPARs regulate the genetic expression involved in fat and carbohydrate metabolism, helping to treat diabetes, high cholesterol, arteriosclerosis, hyper-metabolism and obesity.

> The positive thing about this family of [grapefruit citrus] compounds is that they are non-toxic and can be taken at high doses.
>
> Dr Samuel Wheeler French Jr, liver pathologist, California

Grapefruit: a solid gold superfood

Fresh grapefruit is possibly the most powerful fat-burning fruit anywhere. That is also the power it has in the human body. Grapefruit is one of the healthiest foods to consume for breakfast as it is easy on the digestion, high in fibre, bursting with living enzymatic activity, has prebiotics, is packed with vitamin and plantioxidant components, and naturally burns fat! A grapefruit a day will help to clean out the fat and plaque in your heart in six months. Grapefruit is very powerful, helping to thin the blood, remove plaque and cholesterol from the blood, and burn up drug toxins.

A grapefruit a day will almost certainly keep the doctor away and may prevent heart, bone and constipation problems. Freshly squeezed grapefruit juice is also one of the only foods (alongside melons) that do not require stomach acid for digestion. Stomach acid normally kills enzymes, but with grapefruit juice the enzymes are delivered deep into the intestines. Grapefruit juice is highly alkalising (when fresh) and is a natural cleaning agent that has antiseptic, antibacterial and antifungal properties.

Grapefruit: a treatment for heart disease?

New research from the University of Glasgow's Institute of Molecular, Cell and Systems Biology, published on 12 August 2013 in the *Biochemical Journal*, has identified how molecules that specifically occur naturally in grapefruit may play an important role in the future treatment of heart disease. Many diseases of the circulatory system and heart are directly linked to the improper activation of immune cells, which then stick to the vascular endothelial cells (VECs) that line the blood vessels. Dr Stephen Yarwood noted that the flavanoid naringenin was shown to 'effectively inhibit the inflammatory processes triggered following activation of the receptor for immune molecule IL6 on the surface of VECs. We were surprised to find that flavanoids isolated from citrus fruits were very effective at reprogramming the response of human endothelial cells to immune molecules by switching on genes that exert a natural, "protective" effect against inflammation. Our job now is to find out how flavanoids turn on these protective genes.'

Grapefruit is often free

In New Zealand, most people who have a grapefruit tree on their property don't eat the fruit. When grapefruit season kicks in I go and knock on the door of a house that has a grapefruit tree somewhere on the section. I often take my youngest son, Joel, as he loves grapefruit as much as I do.

We knock on the door and when it's answered, we say very sweetly, 'Hello, we noticed you have a grapefruit tree. We love grapefruit and we were wondering if we could ...' At this stage we are usually interrupted. 'Take as much as you like! I hate those bitter grapefruit!' Brilliant. We can then go and pick fresh grapefruit as we need them, doing a clean-up service for the neighbourhood!

> Eating grapefruit is a process that is similar to the Atkins diet, without many of the side effects. The liver behaves as if fasting, breaking down fatty acids instead of carbohydrates.
>
> Dr Martin L. Yarmush, MD, PhD, Director of the MGH Center
> for Engineering in Medicine, USA

Grapefruit liminoids and bioflavonoids

It is hard to look past grapefruit as part of a fat loss strategy, but remember that only raw grapefruit that includes the white inner skin (the bitter part) offers the complete health benefits. When you eat grapefruit, oranges, lemons or any other citrus fruits, one of the many unique groups of health-promoting compounds you ingest are called citrus liminoids. Liminoids have been shown to help fight cancers of the mouth, skin, lung, breast, stomach and colon. They are another good example and one tiny group of compounds that are present in wholefoods (alongside natural vitamin C) that give effective health benefits but are not present in any man-made synthetic vitamin pills.

Grapefruit strengthens your bones

Grapefruit pulp has been shown to increase bone strength and reduce the risk of osteoporosis. A 248-page report by the Commonwealth Scientific and Industrial Research team concluded that a diet high in citrus offers a 50% risk reduction against mouth, larynx, pharynx and stomach cancer and positive effects for arthritis, asthma, Alzheimer's, Parkinson's disease, macular degeneration, diabetes, gallstones, multiple sclerosis, cholera, gingivitis, optimal lung function, cataracts, ulcerative colitis and Crohn's disease.

Grapefruit and medication

Grapefruit is very effective at thinning the blood and blocking the special enzymes in the wall of the small intestine that can destroy medications and lower drug absorption. For this reason, if you are on prescription medications, please check your drug label warnings before ingesting lots of grapefruit.

Grapefruit and longevity

One of my favourite stories about grapefruit comes from 101-year-old Al Roth. He says, 'Citrus fruit is the secret to longevity.' Mr Roth beat colon cancer at 94 and at 101 reckons he 'will get to 120'. What's his secret? He credits his longevity to citrus. 'Have a fresh orange or grapefruit each day. You're eating one of the best foods possible.'

Celery and weight loss

Celery juice is highly nutritious, incredibly alkalising and one of the most hydrating foods we can put in our bodies. Celery juice is rich in soluble, organic sodium (totally different from table salt), which helps break down any built-up calcium deposits on the joints.

Organic sodium improves nutritional absorption and, as every cell in our body is constantly bathed in a salt solution, the right sodium is very important for long-term health. If the salt level in the human body is not balanced, dehydration occurs. Celery juice is the perfect rehydration drink. The organic potassium/sodium mix in celery juice is a powerful body fluid regulator that stimulates urine production to help rid the body of excess fluid. Special nutrients in the fibre are released during juicing that help bowel movements. This makes celery juice a gentle bowel mover for relieving constipation. As it is highly alkalising, it is very good for building strong bones.

> Juicing is the future of medicine. It cures cancer, reverses heart disease and stabilizes cholesterol and blood pressure. It ends kidney stones and gall stones and reverses depression and psychosis. It builds strong bones and strong muscles. It absolutely reverses type II diabetes in a matter of days, and it obliterates obesity in a matter of weeks.
>
> Mike Adams, nutritionist, editor of *Natural News*

Fasting and exercise

Fasting slows insulin, burns fat and makes you more active. It affects the transcription factor protein-gene-activator called Foxa2. Foxa2 is found in the liver, where it influences fat burning, but also in the hypothalamus, the region of the brain that controls the daily rhythm, sleep, intake of food and sexual behaviour. When you eat, the pancreas releases insulin, which blocks

Foxa2. When you fast, there is a lack of insulin and Foxa2 is active. Fasting lowers the insulin levels in your body so you burn fat for fuel. In the brain, Foxa2 assists the formation of two proteins: MCH and orexin. These two brain-messenger substances trigger the intake of food and increase physical movement. As I mentioned earlier, fasting keeps you active and helps you burn fat. Fasting also causes another SIRT1 enzyme to suppress the activity of a family of proteins called SREBPs, which control fat and cholesterol production.

The Swedish Fast Marches

The famous 1954 Swedish Fast Marches were reported all over the world. Nineteen men fasted while they walked from Gothenburg to Stockholm, a distance of over 520 kilometres, in ten days. Testing showed that the protein level of the blood (serum albumin reading) in the Swedish fast marchers was normal throughout the fasting period, even though they did not eat. No food. Protein levels normal.

While you are fasting your body does what it can to preserve its lean muscularity and body tissue. Dr Lennart Edren, Doctor of Dental Surgery, directed the Swedish Fast Marches. He said, 'This experiment proved to the world the preventive and the therapeutic potentials of fasting.'

> The march clearly showed that man can live for an extended period of time without food, even accomplish a hard physical effort while fasting. The participants felt stronger and had more vigour and vitality after the fast than before it. This was a thorough and objective scientific study of fasting and its prophylactic and therapeutic potentials.
>
> Dr Karl-Otto Aly, participant in Fast Marches

Exercising while fasting

Training while fasting can stimulate adaptations in muscle cells to facilitate and increase energy production through fat burning.[9] When tested, fasting had no negative impact on the speed, power, agility or endurance of athletes.[10] Basically, you burn more body fat when you exercise while fasting than exercising on a stomach filled with carbohydrates.[11] In 1995, after 40 days on water alone, Don Tolman drank one quart of freshly squeezed grape juice and then ran a marathon and was filmed by Hollywood companies Motion Media and the LA Film Factory.

The most push-ups I have ever done without stopping is 160. At the time, I was on the 26th day of a fast. When you fast you save energy and throw the body out of its comfort zone entirely.

The body adapts extremely well to routine. By fasting once a week for a day and then sometimes for three days and then a week or two we provoke the greatest response in our bodies. The body supercompensates with adaptive stress response mechanisms, which augment your resistance to illness and injury, leaving you stronger and healthier.

My amazing son!

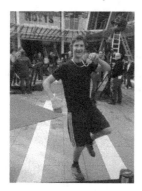 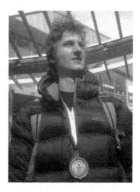

In 2009 our eldest son, Trey, semi-fasted on vegetable juice and green superfoods for 36 hours, then broke a Guinness World Record. He was 20 years old and the event was hopping on a treadmill, a strength and endurance test. He smashed the record by 20 seconds! You can watch the video of him breaking this world record on our website, www.jasonshonbennett.com.

17

The science of fasting

Fasting has been proven to be good for heart disease, cancer treatments, obesity, diabetes, asthma and more. What's not to like?

Jason Shon Bennett

The science behind fasting

Zafar Nomani is a Professor Emeritus of Human Nutrition and Foods at West Virginia University. He is a recipient of the King Hassan II Award from the first International Conference on Scientific and Medical Research on Ramadan. In 2010 he turned 80, and he has fasted regularly since he was a boy. In the early 1980s, he began studying the biochemical and physiological impact of fasting in the US and Pakistan. What he and other researchers discovered was that fasting has clear physical, psychological and social benefits.

Hi Jason, I flew to the UK at end of November, 2011. I decided to try your fasting method to conquer jet lag. And it worked! Most of my family in UK thought I was crazy ('How do you not eat for over 24 hours?'), but I arrived feeling fresher than I usually do and didn't really have jet lag. I drank lots of water and occasional diluted juice. Thanks for the tip. It made my flying trip to UK far more memorable.

Kate on thelifeplan, 2011

Fasting for disease prevention

The Greek Ikarians, longevity champions, observe about 150 days of religious fasting a year. A third of them live into their 90s and beyond in great health and vitality, mostly without drugs or illness. The Hippocrates Institute and Dr Malkmus of Hallelujah Acres have successfully treated thousands of people with fasting and the fresh juice of fruits and vegetables. Naturopathic Doctor Rudolf Breuss used fasting and raw juice therapies successfully on thousands of patients with diseases such as cancer and leukaemia. Positive fasting results are worldwide, long term and phenomenal.

British and German investigators found that the addition of fresh carrot juice or raw spinach juice to the diet of children suffering with severe scurvy resulted in full recovery. A seven- to ten-day fast significantly improves rheumatoid arthritis, and continues to if followed by a healthy vegetarian diet.[1] Fasting improves the 'time adjustment experience' of travelling and beats jet lag.[2] Normally, the body's natural circadian brain-clock dictates when we wake, eat and sleep – all in response to daylight and nightfall. But a second clock takes over when you are fasting, so manipulating this clock can help you adjust to new time zones, faster.[2] While travelling, fasting for about 16 hours is enough. I always fast when travelling long distances.

Fasting and asthma

Asthmatics who fast have fewer symptoms, better airway function and a decrease in the markers of inflammation in the blood.[3] Fasting asthmatic patients have rapid and sustained beneficial effects and lowered symptoms of asthma.[4] I have never had asthmatic symptoms while fasting and I have fasted hundreds of times.

> There has been a general improvement in my asthma,
> it is best when I'm fasting ...
> Antoinette on thelifeplan, 2012

Fasting and cancer

Dr Max Gerson used raw juice therapy in his decades of successful cancer treatments.[5] Cancer treatments are well supported by juice fasting, especially green vegetables, but not water fasting alone. Here is the really interesting thing about normal cells versus cancer cells. All cells, including cancer cells, are fuelled by glucose, which is made from the natural sugars in the healthy carbohydrate foods we eat. When you fast, particularly when you water-only fast, there is no fuel for your normal healthy cells to use, apart from what is stored in and on the body, so the cells either hibernate or switch to the alternate fuel: fatty ketones. Cancerous tumour cells are very different. They lack the ability to turn themselves off, they cannot hibernate, and they cannot use ketones as fuel. Therefore, when you fast and remove glucose, they cannot grow or hibernate, so they die.

Fasting as a support for cancer treatments

Fasting prior to cancer chemotherapy treatment can significantly enhance the cancer-killing effects of the drugs while protecting healthy cells from the side effects and damage.[6] Chemotherapy drugs damage all active and growing cells, whether good or bad. However, when someone fasts healthy cells go into a hibernation-like mode that produces extreme resistance to stress such as chemotherapy. Many specialist cancer doctors suggest juice fasting to give the immune system a break and then to help it better corral the stray cells that escape the initial cancer treatment. Fasting induces a protective shield around healthy cells, allowing them to tolerate a much higher dose of chemotherapy.[7] When fasting, your cells show significant declines in their tendency to divide or proliferate.[8]

In one study, all patients reported fewer side effects when they received chemotherapy while fasting.[9] The effects of the treatment did not alter. In another study, a large group of animals were split into two groups. The first group was given chemotherapy and food and no animals survived the cancer treatments. The second group was given chemotherapy and fasting and **60% of the animals survived**.[10] This is a staggering success rate and one worthy of serious attention from the medical world.

Valter Longo, Director of the Longevity Institute at the University of Southern California, found that a 48-hour fast slowed the growth of five of eight types of cancer in mice. Even better, the effect was stronger the more fasts the animals undertook. Mice with gliomas (very aggressive brain tumors) were more than **twice** as likely to survive if they underwent a two-day fast accompanied by radiation therapy, compared to those that did not have fasting administered.

Lowering the risks

We know that high levels of IGF-1 and glucose in the blood, high insulin levels and being overweight are some of the risk factors for cancer. They are all dramatically and immediately improved by regular fasting. By fasting day three or four, the production of IGF-1 drops to very low levels. By day five, it can drop by as much as 70%. Low levels of IGF-1 are directly associated with a much lower risk of cancer, and an increased lifespan.

Fasting and type II diabetes

Here are a few of the findings from research into fasting and type II diabetes.

▶ We are genetically built for fasting as our insulin regulation improves sevenfold while fasting.[11]

▶ In human trials regular fasting has shown great benefits for those with diabetes.[12]

▶ Fasting can beneficially modulate other indexes of diabetes risk, such as insulin sensitivity.[13]

▶ Fasting one day per week delivers improved insulin sensitivity.[14]

▶ Juice drinkers are generally leaner, and have better insulin sensitivity,[15] which reduces the risk of stroke, heart disease and diabetes.

▶ Juicing helps reduce the risk for diabetes and can help keep weight under control.[16]

▶ Researchers have measured 'improved pancreatic function' and found 'fewer fatty deposits associated with insulin resistance' in those fasting.

Intermittent fasting might achieve much of the benefit seen with bariatric surgery, but without the costs, restriction on numbers and risks associated with surgery. Whether intermittent fasting can be used as a tool to prevent diabetes in those individuals at high risk or to prevent progression in those recently diagnosed with type II diabetes remains a tantalizing notion and we are currently in preparation for clinical trials to assess the effectiveness of this form of lifestyle intervention in various patient groups.

James E. Brown, Michael Mosley and Sarah Aldred, 'Intermittent fasting: a dietary intervention for prevention of diabetes and cardiovascular disease?' *British Journal of Diabetes and Vascular Disease*, April 2013

Fasting on the fresh raw juices of fruits and vegetables, plus vegetable broths and herb teas, results in much faster recovery

from disease and more effective cleansing and rejuvenation
of the tissues than does the traditional water fast.

Dr Otto H. F. Buchinger, who has supervised over 80,000 fasts

Fasting and cardiovascular disease

Hypertension or 'high blood pressure diseases' are the biggest cause and precursor of cardiovascular disease and heart disease death, which kill 40% of all people in the West.[17] So, to lower the devastating death toll from heart disease we need to address its single biggest cause: high blood pressure. At the TrueNorth Health Education Center in California, 174 consecutive hypertensive patients were treated with a plant-based wholefood diet and then a period of fasting.[18] They all started with dangerous blood pressure levels, far higher than 140/90. The results were nothing short of miraculous.

► All patients who started on medication were able to stop medication by the end of the one month programme. This is a **100%** success rate.

► Almost 90% achieved blood pressure less than 140/90 – essentially being cured of their hypertension.

► After six months, all tested patients had an average blood pressure of 123/77.

► This is a **95%** success rate of curing hypertension (and therefore heart disease) with diet and fasting alone.[19]

Fruit juices are the cleansers of the human system, vegetable juices are the builders and regenerators. The juices extracted from fresh raw vegetables and fruits are the means by which we can furnish all the cells and tissues of the body with the elements and the nutritional enzymes which they need, in the manner in which they can be most readily digested and assimilated'

Norman Walker, *The Juice Doctor*, 1970

Fasting and heart disease

Regular fasting protects against heart disease. Krista Varady of the University of Illinois has seen cholesterol level benefits when taking people through fasting. US research cardiologists found that 24-hour fasting can lower the risk of developing coronary artery disease and diabetes and also can improve blood cholesterol levels. In 2007, the American Heart Association's Scientific Sessions revealed that people who fast one day each month have lower rates of heart disease. Those who regularly fast are 45% less likely to be diagnosed with heart disease.[20]

In June 2013 Paul, who is undertaking thelifeplan, emailed me about his experience to date. He said, 'Well, it's now just coming on two months since starting thelifeplan. I've taken part in fasting twice. Both one day fasts. Yesterday I went to my doctor as I needed more medication for my blood pressure. I'm now 85 kg, I started the plan at 91kg. The exciting news: my blood pressure was 180/100; I'm now 148/84. How GOOD is that? I still have further to go but it's so exciting to know I'm on the right track and that I will be able to toss all medication out. Yahoo!'

> I believe that fasting is the 'missing link' in the Western diet. Fasting is one of the best overall healing methods because it can be applied to so many conditions and people. Fasting is the single greatest natural healing therapy. It is nature's ancient, universal remedy for many problems.
>
> Dr Elson Haas, MD, USA

A reversal of heart disease

Fasting for just one day a month causes reduction in clogged arteries by up to 40%.[21] Periodic fasting cuts the risk of heart disease by 58%.[22] Regular fasting significantly lowers blood fat and bad cholesterol and improves cholesterol balance.[23] Fasting renders hard and rusty blood vessels (that cause atheroma) more soft and supple, due to the walls of the blood vessels softening. Blood pressure is reduced while fasting. The blood-clot dissolving fibrinolytic activity of the blood is increased by fasting. Regular fasting halves the death rate of myocardial infarction and lowers the risk of arteriosclerosis and angina pectoris.

Fasting makes the heart younger as the digestive workload is decreased. Apple and purple grape juice help prevent artery hardening.[24] Drinking just 500 ml of beetroot juice a day can substantially reduce blood pressure, lowering your risk of a heart attack.[25] Cholesterol levels drop far more during and after fasting for those who are physically active.[26] The key here is they drop far more than just physical exercise alone. Regular fasting lowers all the 'fat related' coronary heart disease risk indicators.[27]

A 2012 review published in the *British Journal of Diabetes and Vascular*

Disease by a team from Aston University found fasting can limit inflammation, improve levels of sugars and fats in your circulation, cut blood pressure and lower cholesterol levels.

Vegetable juice lowers blood pressure

A small study involving 30 people who drank half a litre of beetroot juice with a little apple juice[28] demonstrated that, for both genders, blood pressure levels dropped six hours after drinking the beetroot juice. In the men the drop was almost five points! Researcher Dr Leah Coles said, 'It's promising that we can see an effect from a single dose. That effect might be even greater over the long term if they are drinking it day upon day.' This is a life-changing result and would equate to **a 10% nationwide reduction in deaths due to heart disease if everyone did it.**

The 2004 INTERHEART study of 30,000 men and women in 52 countries throughout Africa, Asia, Australia, Europe, the Middle East, and North and South America showed that at least 90% of heart disease is lifestyle related.[29] Even in 1961, the mainstream scientific journal, *The American Medical Association* (AMA), said, 'A vegetarian diet can prevent 97% of our coronary occlusions.' This is curing heart disease through simple dietary and lifestyle changes.

In my opinion, a combination of eating a healthy, plant-based wholefood diet, lowering stress, exercising, sleeping well and adopting a routine of Regular Intelligent Fasting® is the solution that could wipe out up to 95% of heart disease worldwide.

thelifeplan®

I have studied enough research and had more than adequate personal experience regarding heart disease being cured through diet for a separate book! However, here I give you a small selection of the results I have had working with people, their doctors, their blood tests and their heart health on thelifeplan.

Yay, I did it! For the first time in my life I fasted the whole day yesterday! I just followed your tips and inspiration and ... success!
I never thought I would ever be able to fast, considering that
I've never before had any willpower where food was concerned, but surprisingly I managed quite well on vegetable juice, green

tea and potato broth. I just kept focusing on why I was doing this. I now feel confident that I can do this again. Thanks for your support and inspiration.

Brenda on thelifeplan, 2012

I had an interesting visit with my GP last Friday. Good news, my total cholesterol is down to 5 (was 5.3), and had good decreases in triglycerides and LDL. The doctor even commented on my nice low pulse rate, and great blood pressure.

Iain on thelifeplan, February 2012

It's been a remarkable journey and life-changing experience for me during the past 14 months on thelifeplan. The programme has totally changed my life and the way I see food and medicine. The programme gave me the tools and knowledge I was missing to heal myself from chronic infections without using medicine or antibiotics. Last month when I visited my GP for a general check-up 'WOF', he was surprised to see my weight, blood pressure, blood results including cholesterol level, and said 'Wow!' In November 2010 my cholesterol reading was 5.5+ and now is below 4, and my blood pressure is normal. I feel great, full of energy, better concentration in my work and studies, my skin is pimple free and I have lost 15 kgs and 10 cm of waist. Thanks for the guidance, advice and wisdom.

Mohammad on thelifeplan, April 2012

I would like to let you know some results I've had. After six weeks on thelifeplan I had to reduce one of my two blood pressure medications by 50% because my blood pressure was so low. I have almost reached my three month goal weight in two months.

Jane on thelifeplan, July 2012

I'm finally off the 7 mark for my cholesterol!! It was nice to read after having been up to 7.4 at one stage in the last three years. My LDL is down .2 and my HDL is up .15. That was good to read so all in all, a happy result with more to come. Thank you for helping me to get back on track.

Anne on thelifeplan, July 2012

Blood pressure with medication was 142/90 six weeks ago. Yesterday I passed medical with no other problems and now it is 134/80!

Gary on thelifeplan, August 2012

My weight on the programme has gone from 76 kg down to 66 kg and now maintaining at 65 kg! My blood pressure is the best it has ever been – from 120/80 down to 112/72! My cholesterol is down from 4.6 to 3.8.

Linda on thelifeplan, August 2012

The doctor insisted that I take 1x cholesterol drug twice a day to bring my levels down to normal range of under 5. My doctor said at my age my cholesterol levels will not come down without medication but will increase as I get older. I made a decision to go the natural route without medication by eating thelifeplan plant-based wholefood diet. Yesterday I went for a cholesterol blood test and got the results this morning from my doctor. My cholesterol levels have come down from 6.1 to 4.5, which is now in normal range. Thank you for bringing my cholesterol levels down naturally without medication.

Valerie on thelifeplan, November 2012

Hi Jason, just a wee update. Working with my doctor I am down to half my statin (10 mg) and no longer take betablockers. I have had a round of blood tests and everything is normal. Happy days! This plant-based wholefood lifestyle really works.

Tom on thelifeplan, May 2013

Dear JSB, I weighed in last Thursday and shed another three kg! Something else that I've noticed – no angina attacks. I used to have a spray for under my tongue, because I would get that horrible intermittent pain, over the past three years, caused by the heart not getting enough oxygen. How fantastic is that! I'm still feeling and looking amazingly well.

Janette on thelifeplan, May 2013

Hi Jason, I had the annual check-up with my GP. He actually asked me if I was on medication because my cholesterol was so good.

Mary on thelifeplan, May 2013

Made it below 64 kg (started at 77 kg) and the good news is that I am completely off high blood pressure tablets, Vit. B12 level is excellent and cholesterol ratio is 2.7 with HDL at 2.02. As you can guess, I am very pleased with myself but really and truly, without the knowledge that you and Tracey have imparted along the way, healthwise, life may have been a very different story. Thank you both so much.

Vicki on thelifeplan, May 2013

You have given me and my family a wonderful tool of fasting. It is a tough job but the results are amazing. The more you do it the more you want it. I have never experienced such a feeling before. I feel as if I am cleaning my internal organs more with every fast. It is just a wonderful simply divine experience! Thank you so much.

Menaka Mahajan on thelifeplan, 2012

Here are my favourite two 'tested by the doctor' results from working with people on their blood pressure, blood cholesterol and blood fat levels.

I finally got up the courage to go and have my medical check-up and blood tests. Results were good. Majority of test results were very normal, including PSA, B12, folate, renal function, iron, diabetic profile (fasting glucose test), complete blood count, C-reactive protein and lipids. My previous results 18 months ago were: cholesterol: 6.1mmol/l, but now it is 4.3mmol/l. Cholesterol and LDL is the lowest they have been in a very long time.

Darryl on thelifeplan, August 2011

My goal was to lower LDL cholesterol by the end of July 2013 when my cholesterol levels would be retested by my doctor. On 21 March 2013 my tested cholesterol levels were 6.3; HDL 1.88, LDL 4.1 and triglyceride 0.8. After being on thelifeplan for three months, my retested results, in July 2013, were

cholesterol 4.9; HDL 1.59, LDL 2.9 and triglyceride 0.9.
I think a reduction in cholesterol from 6.3 to 4.9 is truly
remarkable in such a short time. It endorses what is being taught,
that we are not governed by our genetics! My liver function tests
were excellent and the kidney eGFR (a →90 mL/min. The doctor
said this was 'remarkable' given my age!
As you can imagine, I am pretty excited about the results,
given that the doctor said because of my triglyceride at 0.8, and
that I had not much fat in the diet, I would 'not be able to reduce
the cholesterol'. He recommended I start on statins but agreed to
give me three months without – and look what happened!

Janice, on thelifeplan, July 2013

Fasting and Alzheimer's

The US National Institute on Aging has proved regular fasting helps the brain fight degeneration and recover better from injury. Fasting encourages cellular repair, which leads to higher resistance to Alzheimer's, Parkinson's and the aging process of atrophy. When you fast, the adrenocorticotropic hormone (ACTH, also known as corticotropin), epinephrine and glucagon levels (which stimulate lipolysis and muscle growth) all increase. Both Beta-hydroxy butyrate (BHB) and Human Growth Hormone (HGH) also rise.[30] HGH has shown exponential growth of over 1000% increase while fasting.[31]

BHB is a powerful ketone shown to be beneficial against Parkinson's and Alzheimer's, insulin resistance and free radical damage. HGH is primarily responsible for tissue repair and hypertrophy. When you fast, you get reduced inflammation, and your levels of the inflammatory markers IL-6, C-reactive protein (CRP) and homocysteine all drop.

We know from animal models that if we start an intermittent
fasting diet at what would be the equivalent of middle age in
people, we can delay the onset of Alzheimer's and Parkinson's. If
you look at an animal that's gone without food for an entire day,
it becomes more active. Fasting is a mild stressor that motivates
the animal to increase activity in the brain. From an evolutionary
perspective, this makes sense, because if you are deprived of
food, your brain needs to work harder to help you find something
to eat. The evidence is pretty strong that our ancestors did not

eat three meals a day plus snacks. Our genes are geared to
being able to cope with periods of no food.

Dr Mark P. Mattson, neuroscientist and one of the leading researchers of calorie
restriction at the National Institute on Aging; Professor of Neuroscience,
Johns Hopkins University, USA

The National Institute of Aging fasting studies show a boost in production of a protein called brain-derived neurotrophic factor (BDNF) by up to 400%. This protein helps generate new brain cells and stimulates learning and memory, while protecting brain cells from Alzheimer's and Parkinson's. In a really important aspect to the study, the fasting mice engineered to develop Alzheimer's-like symptoms delayed the onset of memory problems by about six months. This is an incredible result, equivalent to perhaps 20 years' life extension in humans.

Dr Allan Cott, MD, studied the fasting programme of Professor Serge Nikoliav of the Moscow Psychiatric Institute. The programme had a very high success rate for the treatment of chronic refractory schizophrenia with water fasting, without a single fatality, in over 6000 patients. The 2012 studies by the National Institute on Aging, the Longevity Institute at the University of Southern California, the UK's University of Manchester, Intermountain Heart Institute in Murray, Utah, and the University of Illinois all suggest fasting may significantly reduce the risks of developing dementia and mental decline.[32]

Fasting and the immune system

Periodic fasting boosts immunity. Over 80% of your immune system resides in your gut. When there is no food going through the gut, your immune system's workload is greatly reduced. Your immune system is stimulated when fasting, so it more effectively assists in fighting illness and disease. Many enzymes from raw fruits and vegetables are used by our digestive system for food metabolism, and they also feed and strengthen the immune system. Unfortunately, these enzymes are destroyed when heated above 50°C and some plant nutrients are 'locked up' with the fibre content of the food, making it harder for those with weakened digestive systems (from eating the modern diet) to access the goodies in them.

This is another area where fasting is effective. Juicing fruits and vegetables allows the body to consume large amounts of natural nutrients in an easy to absorb manner. Fasting with freshly made juices gives better absorption of these super-healthy natural xanthophyll carotenoids and beneficial plant compounds.[33]

Last week I caught a cold. The next day came the sinus and headache (typical headcold stuff). So, I thought I'd approach this one differently. Took the next day off work and fasted. Took a second day off work, was going to fast again but feeling much better than the previous day, ate, but only small portions. By the third day went back to work feeling cold had completely gone, minus a bit of mucus. One more good sleep and I was 100% again. A three day recovery from a cold in me is unheard of. In the past a cold used to last up to two weeks (despite taking multiple packets of Day & Night flu tablets and multi-vitamins). I definitely believe the fasting, good rest and continual good nutrition were the major points to such a quick recovery in me, especially without the use of any drugs whatsoever.

Steve on thelifeplan, 2013

Fasting and fertility

It is a very simple process: less food means less free radical damage means less aging. Fasting has been shown to prolong the reproductive lifespan.[34] Basically, if you do not have enough calories over an extended time frame, the body closes down the reproductive area. Once normal food conditions resume, the conserved stem cells can produce a brand new crop of sex cells, complete with youthful and fertile eggs. A study on worms (worms and humans share many genes and traits) revealed that extremely old worms on a restricted diet, could generate new eggs and produce healthy offspring long after their normally fed counterparts had reproduced and died. If you have infertility problems, you might consider fasting one day per week for a few months while eating a nutritious, plant-based wholefood diet. Then try to conceive. When you are fasting you have a huge lowering in oxidative stress. People who live to be 100 years old have lower levels of oxidative stress than those who live to be 70.

Just want to thank you for getting my life back. I now have endless amounts of energy, I am fitter than I have ever been, and surfing better than I ever have in 30 years. I feel incredible.

My sleep has improved out of sight. At 132 kg my goal was to get to 90 kg, and I am now happily at 72 kg. My wife and I had been trying to fall pregnant for six years. We were going to start IVF this year, however, three months into thelifeplan we fell pregnant naturally. Our first baby is due in three weeks! Also, I've been a mild asthmatic all my life and that also disappeared halfway through thelifeplan, and I have not had an attack since.

Steve on thelifeplan, Queensland, Australia, November 2013

Juice fasting

Raw fresh juices, as well as freshly made vegetable broths, are rich in super nutrition. Juice fasting can be done with one juice or many. For a first fast, I recommend fruit juices in the mornings (cleansing) and vegetable juices in the afternoon or evening (healing). However, vegetable juice alone is the ultimate option.

Fruit juices can include any fruit you like! The addition of freshly made vegetable and fruit juices to the diet gives excellent results in cases of malnutrition (which most of us are suffering from). You can mix the pulp back into the juice if you genuinely require more fibre, as this will help with beneficial bacteria levels and waste elimination.

It is helpful to have a good quality pre-made juice back-up while fasting, in case you run out of time to make your own fresh juices. My favourite New Zealand pre-made juice is 100% pure dark purple grape juice made by Greenways. Purple grape juice has the highest phenolic content of the commonly found juices. Purple grape juice has been shown to improve heart health, lower LDL oxidation levels and is a powerful vasodilator (dilates and opens the walls of blood vessels). Basically, use 100% pure juices if you are buying them, and water them down before drinking.

Juices have living nutrients that are absorbed very quickly for instant energy, cell regeneration and detoxification, all without taxing the digestive system. Freshly made juice provides a synergistic natural complex of living enzymes, minerals, vitamins, natural plantioxidants, trace elements and soluble fibre. For example, a regular glass of carrot juice contains five grams of protein, 35 mg of vitamin C and 100,000 IU of betacarotene, alongside another 20–30 health enhancing and immune strengthening carotenoids and polyphenols.

Juicing and chlorophyll

Juicing is the single best way to get living chlorophyll into your body. Chlorophyll is the green colour in plants and is one of the most powerful natural medicines that exists. Chlorophyll is basically 'stored sunlight' in the form of biophotons. We eat the plant and convert this energy into glycogen to fuel our muscles. Chlorophyll increases the flow of oxygen to all parts of the body, enabling us to release more carbon dioxide, toxins and stress. Why is this important?

▶ High oxygen levels → an aerobic environment → disease cannot live.

▶ Low oxygen levels → an anaerobic environment → disease thrives.

> Fasting cures disease, dries up bodily humors, puts demons to flight, gets rid of the impure thoughts, makes the mind clear, and the heart pure, and the body sanctified, and raises humanity ...
>
> Atheneus, an ancient Greek physician

Juice fasting cleans the entire system

My favourite fruit juice mix is 60% orange and 10% each of kiwifruit, strawberry, lime and lemon. It has an absolutely stunning, crisp, fresh, tart flavour with a tasty bite. I call that particular drink 'The Tracey' (after my beautiful wife). Plain watermelon with a squeeze of lemon is straight from heaven.

My favourite vegetable juice mix is 60% celery, 10% carrot, cucumber and beetroot with some ginger. The last part is a small amount of any other strong healing herbal bitters thrown in for added zing – parsley, dandelion or alfalfa is very beneficial and helpful. Romaine lettuce is one of the best green vegetables you can juice. You can also juice other types of lettuce, such as red or green lettuce. For variety, try adding large handfuls of kale, Swiss chard, collard greens or bok choy.

The positive effects continue for up to 24 hours after drinking your favourite fresh juice. Just throw a mix of your favourites into a juicer and experiment! The bottom line is that vegetable juicing alone has the most therapeutic benefits and this is what I stick to now while fasting: vegetables and water.

Juices, your kidneys and your bladder

Carrots, cucumbers and beetroot cleanse the kidneys very well. Add garlic as this will ensure a balance of beneficial nutrients (while avoiding excess sugars, such as may occur with carrot or fruit juices alone).

The bladder is like a storage bag, with 90% of bladder cancers occurring along the inner lining (the epithelium). If this tissue is regularly soaked by acidic, toxic urine, there is damage. Remember, 'Healthy pee helps keep you disease free!' Soak the inside of your bladder and large intestine with the leftover alkaline charged water from vegetable juices and help prevent all forms of bladder disease.

In 2003, 79-year-old British granddad Ray Wiseman was diagnosed with severe bladder cancer[35] and was not expected to survive. Ray started each day with a glass of fresh broccoli juice. In 2008, scans revealed that the cancer had stopped spreading and his chances of a full recovery were high. Ray attributed the turnaround in his condition to the daily broccoli juice.

WARNING! Fasting shows up your food addictions

When we are mad, upset, stressed, lonely, irritated, frustrated, grouchy, tired, heartbroken or just plain bored, what do we usually do? We eat. What we eat is the problem. If we pigged out on celery stalks then that would be a good thing. However, what we eat is anti-nutrient, rubbish food that gives us a quick fix of highly acidic sugar, salt, fat, gluten, chocolate or caffeine. These foods feed the emotional cycle, which is why junk food sells so well. I used to go for chocolate afghans or coconut chocolate: thick, fatty and sweet – yum! Regular Intelligent Fasting® is one of the best ways to beat and change your food addictions.

18
Preparation for fasting

Fasting is part of my long-term view on healing the human body. It is not a quick fix, a 'one-off' type treatment. It is part of a healthy and balanced choice to protect yourself from preventable modern lifestyle diseases.

Jason Shon Bennett

WARNING

If any of the following conditions describes you: underweight, undernourished, obese, very overweight, pregnant, lactating, blood sugar problems, hypoglycemia, diabetes, liver or kidney disease, overly hypochondriacally focused, have an eating disorder, or suffering any other systemic disease, such as cancer or a serious heart condition, or if you are under 18 years old, consult your chosen health professional before fasting. This is a thorough and cautious list, but it does need to be pointed out that fasting while in expert hands is always best.

> A little starvation can really do more for the average sick man
> than can the best medicines and the best doctors.
>
> Mark Twain

Fasting can be a highly emotional experience

The one thing that many people underestimate about fasting is the emotional journey. As most of us eat for our emotional state (instead of our body) we can experience irrational and erratic feelings while fasting. The impulse to snack is all in the mind, so don't go blaming your biology.

Fasting can leave you feeling highly emotional and cranky in the short term because it takes time for your body to break those long-lived psychological or biological habits. When you are fasting you cannot stuff those feelings back down because the foods are not in your stomach to suppress them. Be mentally prepared. When you fast, you can't hide out and you can't stuff food in, so you can become a highly emotional, whiny, grumpy, moody pain-in-the-butt!

Warn your friends and family if you are trying fasting for the first time!

Cravings

If food cravings arose biologically then people all over the world would get the urge for similar foods in response to nutritional needs. Yet there are huge cross-cultural differences in the kind of foods we crave.

There is no scientific evidence that food cravings are linked to nutritional deficiencies in any way at all. Cravings are not the body telling us we 'need' a vitamin or mineral because it is missing from our diet and somehow needs replacing. If this was genuinely the case, we would crave fruit and vegetables every day! Food cravings are emotionally and psychologically driven[1] and most comfort food cravings are a response to stress.[2] Stress and emotional upheaval stimulate a flood of hormones and emotions that prompt pleasure-seeking eating patterns, such as pigging out on chocolate and ice cream.[3]

A new relationship with food

Fasting is a rebooting of the body systems. Fasting frees you from the tyranny of food and gives you a different appreciation of time and energy. Fasting encourages you to rethink your eating habits.

When you fast you will be stunned at how many times you habitually reach for food. Watching television, feeling stressed or bored, when you are travelling, and so on: you reach for food in all sorts of circumstances that have nothing to do with hunger.

It's enlightening to become aware of your attitudes towards food and eating. We have deep emotional connections with food, which are often revealed during a fast. Fasting therefore develops your inner will power and strengthens your mind to master hormones produced during times of stress, anger, desire or weakness.

> I often observe in the fasting participants that by four days of fasting, concentration seems to improve, creative thinking expands, depression lifts, insomnia stops, anxieties fade, the mind becomes more tranquil and a natural joy begins to appear. It is my hypothesis that when the physical toxins are cleared from the brain cells, mind-brain function automatically and significantly improves and spiritual capacities expand.
>
> Dr Gabriel Cousins, MD, psychiatrist, California

Time alters while fasting

One of the coolest things about fasting is the amount of extra time you get. It is wonderful. Time seems to slow, so if you feel you never have enough time for anything, then you will find fasting completely alters this perception. You do not have to prepare breakfast, lunch, dinner or snacks, so all that time (two to three hours each day) becomes available. You can read more, do things that have been put off for ages, visit people, and so on. You make your daily juice mix and off you go!

Fasting is refreshing to mind, body and soul. During and after fasting, your personal experience of your body, your spirituality and creativity, as it were, is vastly enhanced and elevated. This alone is worth the experience. You sleep less, you are more awake, you are more alive. You are hungrier for life!

Hunger

Do not fear hunger, nothing but good will come of it. The greatest musicians, artists and leaders always did their best work when they were 'still hungry'. The best piece of advice actor Morgan Freeman ever gave to Samuel L. Jackson was to 'stay hungry'.

Limbic hunger refers to the limbic system of the brain, which is where your instinctive behaviors reside. Somatic hunger means 'of the body' or the sensation of 'tummy rumbling'. When you fast for more than three days this alters, and you really start to see how little food you actually need. Don't worry, your body's hunger cycle ultimately adjusts. When you are fasting, ignore the hunger pangs and they will subside within 30–45 minutes as the body begins to break down some of its stored fats for energy.

Almost everyone can fast

As a general rule, the more toxic you are when you start a fast, the worse you may feel. If you have been overeating, living on junk foods, eating lots of processed meats and dairy products, or using pharmaceutical drugs, you should go very slowly with fasting and, for your first time, attempt only one day. If you eat mostly healthy foods, fasting is surprisingly no big deal and can often be a pleasant experience.

Expect good moments and bad ones while fasting. I have watched people on their first fast glide through effortlessly, full of energy and vitality, feeling exhilarated and liberated. I have watched others lose body heat, get headaches, fatigue, nausea, excess mucous, symptoms of influenza or a cold, and experience perspiration, hunger pangs, bad breath, dark urine, skin eruptions, dizziness, nausea, palpitations, muscle pains, cramps, diarrhoea, flatus, irregularities of the heart, increased body odour and a tongue that takes on a concentrated furriness, not to mention the extreme emotions!

> In normal health subjects, moderate fasting, maybe one day a week, or cutting back on calories a couple of days a week, will have health benefits for almost anybody.
>
> Dr Mark P. Mattson, Professor of Neuroscience,
> Johns Hopkins University, USA

These are the main points to remember before and during your fast.

▶ Fasting is generally safe for everyone who is well.

▶ The healthier you are, the longer you can fast.

▶ Stay relaxed as much as you can, and get plenty of rest during a fast.

▶ Eat good, healthy, fresh food for at least a week before fasting.

► You can experience discomfort when initially cleaning out your diet, especially in the first few days of weaning off refined sugar and flour. These symptoms generally disappear by day three. This is your accumulated waste moving into the bloodstream for removal.

► You generally lose your appetite four days into a fast.

► Some people can continue to work as normal right through a long sustained fast, others need to rest and sleep all day.

► You may find that skin rashes or pimples appear. This will pass.

► Be gentle with yourself. Take the basics from my fasting regime and mould them into a fast that suits you and your body. If spirulina works for you but not barley grass, then just have spirulina. If you hate apple cider vinegar but you crave a little lemon juice, use the lemon juice.

Fasting is not an exact science. We are all different people with different biochemical systems, DNA, genetics, digestive systems, food histories and exercise regimes. Trial and error and success and failure are all part of the process.

19

How to fast regularly and intelligently

Regular Intelligent Fasting® is the miracle cure.

Jason Shon Bennett

Recommended ingredients for a successful fast

▶ A good, strong juicer.

▶ Two cups of linseed, one cup of pumpkin seeds, one cup of sunflower seeds, one cup of almonds and one cup of sesame seeds. Mix these and store in a jar. This is the seed/nut mix I mention in the fasting instructions later in this chapter.

▶ Lots of fresh, seasonal fruits and vegetables.

▶ Fresh ginger and fresh lemons for making warm ginger tea/water.

▶ Ice blocks for a treat while fasting. You can pre-juice fresh grapefruits or use other great enzyme rich fruits, then freeze.

▶ Spirulina, barley grass and chlorella tablets and/or powder. A good option is all three blended as a powder.

▶ A good variety and supply of natural and pure herbal teas. Any flavour you like, but make sure they are 100% natural. Good choices for their medicinal powers are dandelion, nettle, liquorice and peppermint.

▶ Aloe vera juice (high quality, inner-gel juice only).

▶ Good quality apple cider vinegar that contains 'mother culture'.

▶ A psyllium husks mixture, ideally containing prebiotics, probiotics, digestive enzymes and slippery elm. You get plenty of fresh soluble fibre while fasting but less insoluble fibre, hence the psyllium.

▶ A loofah or body scrubbing glove of some sort. This helps to shift dry, dead-surface skin cells as well as stimulate circulation in the lumpy thigh and buttocks region!

> Man is the only animal who persists in eating when he is sick, even though he may have no appetite and food makes him nauseous. Fasting is a calming experience. It is restful. It relieves anxiety and tension. It is rarely depressing and it is often downright exhilarating.
>
> Dr Alan Cott, MD, *Fasting: The Ultimate Diet*

Tips for fasting

▶ Have a goal when fasting: plan for it and prepare for it.

▶ Go into a fast already fit so you can carry on exercising while fasting. Your ability to lift and exercise your own body weight will increase incredibly, but go easy on the free weights workouts.

▶ I recommend starting with a one-day fast on either a Saturday or Sunday when you can be at home. If it goes well, two weeks later try fasting for the entire weekend. Then a month or so later, try three days. The first fast is usually the most mentally challenging.

▶ If it doesn't go well, don't beat yourself up. Draw a line in the sand and try again the following week, and keep trying until you complete your full one-day fast. You will get there.

▶ Subsequent fasts get easier as you progressively get healthier and your body has less accumulated toxins to deal with. Build to longer fasts slowly over a year or so, as long as they continue to be beneficial to you.

▶ Relax, do not be too rigid, go to bed early and get enough sleep.

▶ You may get a little testy while fasting as we eat junk foods out of boredom, habit or emotional need. Chocolate, chips and lollies give us an immediate lift and an immediate drug-like feeling of happiness (which is why they sell so well). Watch your emotions carefully because you will be more prone to being snappish and irritable.

► Drink as much as you feel the need to, but do not drink until you feel bloated. Initially you will be drinking all day, but you will find the longer you fast the less liquid you need. Trust your instincts when it comes to water intake. There is no set amount for juice in a day, just what feels healthy and comfortable for you. While fasting, I usually have between 2–4 glasses of freshly made vegetable juice over a day.

► Dress warmly. You get colder as your body fat reserves fall.

► During fasting, before you stand up, take one or two deep breaths to get the heart pumping and to stop light-headedness.

► Do not use harsh laxatives. They are for emergency use only.

► Use the loofah or bodyglove scrubber before your shower or bath as you are shedding lots of skin cells and toxins through the skin.

► Always have a support person who knows what you are doing and why, so they can help when you feel low and encourage you when you need it. Flatmates, family or workmates are the best support people.

► Fasting with a friend is the best fasting of all.

► Stick with foods you are used to eating such as good healthy vegetable juices. Do not try any unusual or new foods on a fast as foods that may cause a reaction will be amplified while fasting. Once you have fasted successfully a few times, add the supergreen foods if you like.

► Your breath may smell really bad. This is a result of the blood cleaning toxins from the body and your bowel letting go of old rotting waste. Carry a toothbrush and toothpaste with you at all times!

You will not only feel revitalized, but also will look younger than before fasting. This is not only because of lost pounds but mostly because fasting has such a rejuvenating effect on all the vital internal organs, including the functions of the all important endocrine glands, which are so decidedly responsible for how young or how old you feel and look.

Paavo O. Airola, Naturpathic Doctor, PhD, Canada

> The body gives back when you go without.
>
> Jason Shon Bennett

The 'eat whatever you like, then fast' diet

Let me make it perfectly clear that I **do not** agree with the latest 'eat whatever you like and then fast' diets. The entire point of fasting, and all the historical evidence about it working, is based on eating well and making other dietary and lifestyle changes – as well as fasting. An example of why I am no fan of the current trend of fasting books can be illustrated using some of the comments and advice given by one of the authors of this book. In an interview he said, 'Milk, eggs, butter, bacon … is always in my fridge' and, 'I am in France at the moment, so I had a croissant and some cheese with a big mug of coffee for breakfast', and 'My favourite junk food is hamburgers'. In my opinion, none of this is good advice if you are regularly fasting, you are wanting to improve bowel health, increase regularity, clean the liver, and are seeking to lower your risk of heart disease, liver disease, breast cancer, bowel cancer, diabetes or obesity. Regular Intelligent Fasting® is best done alongside healthy dietary and lifestyle changes – not junk food, refined pasties, processed meat and coffee.

When you use RIF you will look after yourself while fasting by getting enough sleep, managing your stress levels, and making smart lifestyle changes such as not smoking or drinking (or drinking only in moderation at times of social celebration). Fasting is a support strategy used in your healthy lifestyle, not a magic bullet to junk-food consumption.

When you are not fasting, you eat a healthy, balanced, plant-based wholefood diet. Eating 600 calories or a hamburger while fasting is **not** fasting. Nor is it intelligent or healthy. As written in the *Essene Science of Fasting*, 'There are some kinds of fasts which must be wholly condemned: fasts which are only inspired by the wish to follow a system momentarily in vogue.'

The Fast-Master's Master-Fast

Following over 25 years of regular fasting, here is my most effective, energising, cleansing and rejuvenating fast. It has been followed and completed by a vast number of people all over the world, for anything from 1–40 days. It is suitable for first-time fasters and experienced fasters alike.

The night before

Soak three tablespoons of the nut/seed mixture mentioned earlier in a full glass of lightly sea-salted water. Mix well. The sprinkle of sea salt is optional and only there to help break down the seeds hard cell walls.

On waking

In the morning, drink or sip one glass of warm water, with 1 or 2 tablespoons of pure inner-gel aloe vera juice, 1 or 2 tablespoons of apple cider vinegar and a squeeze of fresh lemon juice. You can have any amount of each of these, or only one, or just plain water if you like. The apple cider vinegar is there to stimulate the digestion, get things moving, balance the pH and replenish gut bacteria. For those who are bloated, the aloe vera is the best stomach 'calmer' I have come across. The lemon juice is included for its alkalising effects.

Gently exercise

Walk, run, skip, swim – whatever is your thing, but get your heart beating for at least 40 minutes (more if you feel inspired). When I fast I do push-ups, handstands, yoga and a 90-minute daily walk. Make sure you warm down and gently stretch afterwards.

Massage

Massage your tummy to stimulate the colon to remove faecal matter that may be stuck to the walls of your bowels. Do this while lying down.

Breakfast

Slowly chew and swallow the nut/seed drink you made the night before. Be prepared as this has quite an unusual taste and consistency, but it provides you with all the essential fatty acid oils the body needs each day. If you are exercising or working, then you can also take up to 10 grams of pure spirulina in tablet or powder from. Brush your teeth and sip on pure water or pure herbal teas as desired. The nut/seed mix and the supergreens are optional.

Lunch

Make a fresh vegetable juice (or go to a juice bar if you can't make it at home or work). Make it heavy on the greens. The ideal would be 60% greens (celery, kale, spinach, cabbage, cavolo nero, dandelion leaves), 20% cucumber, and 10% each of carrot and beetroot. Add 2 heaped tablespoons of green superfoods of your choice (for example, spirulina, chlorella, barley grass or wheat grass) if you would like the extra energy and benefits they deliver.

Ginger is also great for warming the body and removing toxins and poisons. Sip this vegetable juice all day as you feel like it, or just treat it like breakfast and then lunch with just water in-between.

Take no fizzy drinks, sports drinks, energy drinks, alcohol, coffee or black tea of any sort. If you are really feeling the sugar cravings, make up a fresh fruit juice of locally grown seasonal fruits. Freshly squeezed grapefruit juice is best of all. If you can't make it fresh, use the best quality organic dark grape juice you can find. I recommend Greenways in New Zealand. You can add a green superfoods mixture to it if you like. Then brush your teeth.

Another option is to make one big vegetable juice in the morning and sip it throughout the day, as required when hungry or thirsty, without anything else.

Storage

You can store freshly made juice in the fridge for up to 24 hours, with only a moderate nutritional loss if it is in a sealed glass container. Make sure the juice has minimal oxygen levels by filling the container to the top, and then squeeze a half lemon into it.

Dinner

Mix two tablespoons of the psyllium husks mixture into a large glass of water and drink it immediately (it grabs 25 times its weight in water and thickens up very quickly). A tablespoon of slippery elm powder in water is also very beneficial for reducing body acidity. This is particularly good for those wanting to clean out the intestines.

After dinner

Simmer a vegetable broth made of chopped potatoes (and sweet potatoes or others if you like) with skins on. You can add a sprinkle of natural sea salt if you wish. Strain the juice and drink it throughout the evening. This is a tasty, mineral-rich broth that is a fantastic source of calcium, potassium and other minerals. It nourishes and strengthens your bones like few other foods can; it is a bone-builder alongside the celery juice.

At night

If you are fasting again the next day, soak three tablespoons of the nut/seed mixture mentioned earlier in a full glass of lightly sea-salted water. Mix it well.

Repeat for as many days as you like, but remember, I always recommend starting with just one day for your first fast.

> The bottom line is that it [fasting] is the only thing that's ever really been shown to prolong life. Ultimately, aging is a product of a high metabolic rate, which in turn increases the number of free radicals we consume. If you stress the body out by restricting calories or fasting, this seems to cause it to adapt and slow the metabolism down. It's a version of 'what doesn't kill you makes you stronger'.
>
> Dr Michael Mosley, UK, 2012

Additional fasting tips

► Remove all temptation. Hide it at the back of the fridge or cupboard, lock it in a safe and throw away the key, whatever you need to do!

► Set your goals for the day and write them down somewhere you can look at when you need inspiration. Why are you doing this, what do you want to achieve, how will it make you feel?

► Keep yourself busy. Start a project you've been meaning to do, write a letter to a friend/family member, go for a walk around the block, watch a movie, do the washing or vacuuming, have a rest with a book.

► Try not to think about food – change your thoughts as soon as your mind wanders to the kitchen.

► If you feel hungry, get busy away from food temptations such as the fridge or pantry.

► Lunchtime can be one of the greater challenges of the fasting day, especially if you can smell food. Take yourself away from temptation and go for a gentle walk outside if you can. This is a good time to have a big glass of revitalising vegetable juice, or perhaps some hot water and ginger for the water fasters.

The key to successful fasting? Enjoy yourself! You are challenging your body physically and your mind mentally. You are doing something most people will never even consider. Enjoy that feeling!

If you are nearly there but are tempted to eat, think of the seven Rs:

| 1. Rest | 2. Recover | 3. Rebuild | 4. Refresh |
| 5. Rejuvenate | 6. Revitalise | 7. Reboot. | |

Repeat these every time you feel like relenting. Remember some of the reasons you are fasting, such as:

▶ to become focused and ready for a big project/task/event ahead

▶ to improve clarity and concentration for a busy day at work

▶ to give the digestive system a break

▶ to give the liver a big clean out

▶ to improve skin

▶ to feel more energised and lighter

▶ to regain control over how and what you're eating

▶ to break naughty habits

▶ to heighten senses.

> Every fool can fast, but only the wise man
> knows how to break a fast.
>
> George Bernard Shaw

How to end a fast successfully

Signals that the cleansing process is coming to an end are when your tongue clears up and your breath is naturally fresh. Break your fast with something like a grapefruit. Do not overeat. Eat light, healthy foods such as salads and fruits. Do not overeat. Soups are a great way to introduce food again. Do not overeat. Avoid heavy foods such as meat and dairy products for a week or so (or for the rest of your life, as I strongly recommend). Do not overeat.

Eating after fasting

When you fast and then you eat again, if you suddenly get a runny nose, or start sneezing or have short breath or an asthma attack, it becomes very clear the food you have just ingested has an immediate impact on your health.

I have a bivalve seafood allergy and the reactions are violent: vomiting, sweating, body ache and instant sleepiness. I also have food intolerances that include gluten and dairy foods. If I have just ingested foods containing gluten (such as bread or cakes) or dairy products for more than three days in a row, I get a mixture of the following symptoms: tiredness, a thick head on waking, sneezing and mucous in the nose, sticky messy poos, bloating, cold sores, sore joints, tightness in the chest, itchy eyes, constipation, pimples around my chin, and dry lips. I also get a streaming nose and the sneezes if I spend more than an hour near a cat in a closed room. If I experience all of the above, my asthma comes back with a vengeance. Fasting was a critical part in clarifying this and healing my illness for good.

FAST: Feel Amazing, Stimulate Transformation!

Give your body a regular break. Get on the FAST track to health. Fasting leads to a more effective and broadly enhanced physiological function. This is much like finally getting a chance to clean under the bed, in the closet and out in the garage, leading to an immaculate, brand new, recharged, clear, fully functional and spacious living environment. Fasting enables you to Rest, Recover, Rebuild, Refresh, Rejuvenate, Revitalise and Reboot.

Fasting is fantastic! You feel amazing, you function better and fly higher. Your bowels flow easier (this is a fact)!

If you fast for one day each week for seven years, you will have fasted for one entire year. If you also fast for two weeks every quarter, after seven years you will have fasted for almost two years. It's been estimated that if humans fasted just one day each week, they would live twice as long!

Fasting is one of those things you must do at least once in your life.

Water fasting

Water fasting is **not** for beginners. I do not recommend water fasting until you have mastered regular, green superfood fasting, consistently and easily. Juice fasting, for most people, is far better in many ways. **Do not** attempt water fasting until you have mastered juice fasting. Juice fasting is the first step; over time you can extend the periods on water alone while juice fasting.

Water fasting may lead to dizziness and blackouts. Water fasting is the pinnacle of fasting in the sense that the body gets a total rest. When you water fast, without any sugar intake of any kind, your blood sugar remains at baseline and the body has no need of insulin, so those levels are minimal and insulin sensitivity is improved. Blood insulin levels drop dramatically and stabilise effectively during the first 24 hours of fasting.

Water fasting is more unusual and intense than juice fasting as you do not have to do anything. You do not go to the fridge, you do not make juices, and you do not need to remember anything at all about your intake. You just sip water.

This is a really strange situation for your brain, because you will walk to the fridge or pantry on automatic pilot. It demonstrates in the clearest possible way how much you overeat; how many times you habitually reach for food or heavily flavoured drinks.

Remember, the point of fasting is not to be miserable or to focus on being hungry, but to retrain our bodies and strengthen our minds by saying 'no' for a while. On a water fast it is fine to have a grated ginger simmered in a pot of water (or another comparable drink) to boost circulation and to keep you warm.

> There's no question in my mind that a water-only fast, conducted with proper preparation and supervision, is the most effective way to burn up unwanted adipose tissue and eliminate stored toxins. But to do a water-only fast properly, it's best to rest around the clock, both physically and emotionally, and to fast for at least a week. To engage in everyday activities while consuming nothing but water is a good way to quickly lose skeletal muscle mass, which, for a number of reasons, isn't good for your health.
>
> Dr Ben Kim, USA

In accomplishing a fast, you will realise three very important things

1. YOU DIDN'T DIE! Most people have enough spare calories to go 40 days without eating.

2. You strengthened your self discipline and inner-confidence. You accomplished something that most people will never do. This is a milestone accomplishment in self-control.

3. You observed yourself and recognised when you habitually reach for food. This helps reform your paradigm on food and your eating habits.

Go you!

> The skin becomes more youthful during fasting. The eyes clear up and become brighter. One looks younger. The visible rejuvenation

in the skin is matched by manifest evidences of similar but
invisible rejuvenescence throughout the body.

Herbert Shelton, water fasting overseer, USA

A long term aim: Regular Intelligent Fasting®

RIF recommends fasting for one day most weeks and one week in 12. However, on your journey the ultimate aim is to get used to fasting. Each time you progressively take in less, you get closer to being able to fast on water alone. I can now regularly water-fast for one to six days. What fasting taught me was that I had been regularly eating foods that kept me weak, clogged my digestive system, constipated me and stressed my immune system (so it was unable to protect me).

I realised that it was not in my best interests to eat foods containing gluten, dairy produce, meat and bivalve seafood. They all weakened me and kept me sick. Okay, so be it. I came to terms with having the body I have, and it does not like these foods. I stopped eating them and my health took another giant step forward. The bloating stopped, the cold sores stopped. The asthma stopped and the sneezing stopped.

Golden Rule No. 2: Regular Intelligent Fasting®

I realised that after years of poor food choices, sickness and drugs, I had totally stripped my intestines of good bacteria and gut flora. I had lots of rebuilding to do. I was also emptying my bowels only once a day. With this in mind I started studying the bowels. This was when I learned that the digestive system is the single most important part of the human body and the critical key to your health, vitality and longevity.

Fasting, lifestyle changes and eating a plant-based wholefood diet are the key elements in transforming your bowel and digestive health. Transforming your bowel and digestive health is the single most important thing you can do for your health long term.

You will not give even an hour's rest to me, your stomach.
Day after day, every hour you keep on eating.
You have no idea how I suffer, O trouble-making ego.
It is impossible to get on with you.

Osborne

Appendix A
Centenarians tell their secrets

I'm seeing 100-year-olds who are not only 100 years old but in great shape. They're driving and painting, and they say life is beautiful. I have this bias that makes me believe we have the ability as a species to get to 100 if we prevent some of these age-related diseases. The cost of treating 100-year-olds in their last two years of life is a third of what it costs to treat somebody aged 70 to 80. People who die between 70 and 80 are sick in the last few years of their life. Centenarians are dying healthy, all of a sudden.

Professor Nir Barzilai, Albert Einstein College of Medicine, New York

If you want to know how to live a long and healthy life, ask someone who has lived a long and healthy life. Don't ask an overweight, pre-diabetic, cholesterol-ridden, 50-year-old alcoholic doctor what it takes to live to 100 years old. That doctor has no idea and will not get to 100. Instead, ask a bunch of healthy 100-year-olds who do not need to visit the doctor.

Keep a quiet heart, sit like a tortoise, walk sprightly like a pigeon and sleep like a dog.

Li Qing Yun, an ancient centenarian

The oldest person ever

According to the official world record books, the oldest person ever verified was Frenchwoman Jeanne Calment. Born in 1875, she met Vincent Van Gogh when she was 14, and died in 1997 at the age of 122. When a reporter asked on her 120th birthday if she felt he would be seeing her again on her 121st, she replied, 'I see no reason why not; you look healthy enough to me.' Her secrets were, among other things, 'Garlic, vegetables, and I poured olive oil over everything I ate ...'

The world's oldest man was Jiroemon Kimura, who was born on 19 April 1897 and died on 12 June 2013. He turned 116 years old in 2013 and is officially the oldest recorded man in history.[1] When he was born, life expectancy in Japan was 44 years. He says his secret was a strict, healthy plant-based diet of rice, vegetables, miso soup, porridge, red beans and fish. He did not smoke and rarely drank alcohol. His secret was 'to eat three small meals per day, and to stop eating when the stomach is about 80% full.' He survived famine periods saying, 'eat light to live long'. He was a postman for more than 40 years (walking all day most days), during a period marked by food shortages that caused malnutrition. He still had normal blood pressure at age 116. Every year he celebrated his birthday with rice, pumpkins and sweet potatoes, happily prepared by his 60-year-old grandchildren!

RIP, Jiroemon. Even though I never met you, I have followed your fantastic exploits for many years. You have always inspired me. You taught me the simple, common sense that I now pass to others. You were disciplined and strongly committed to living right and eating well. An inspiration to many of us, you walked the talk and lived a long healthy life free of drugs and disease.

> Stay active and eat right.
>
> Maria Suarez, 100-year-old mother of nine,
> who takes no medication and grows her own vegetables

Li Qing Yun

Li Qing Yun was a Chinese medicine physician, herbal expert, qigong master and tactical consultant. He was reputed to have lived for 256 years, from 1677–1933 (obviously not proven). What were his secrets? He went to bed early, got up early and meditated regularly. He did not drink hard liquor or smoke, and ate his vegetarian meals at regular times while enjoying wolfberry (goji berry) tea. In his May 1933 obituary published in *Time* magazine, his final advice was to, 'keep a quiet heart, sit like a tortoise, walk sprightly like a pigeon and sleep like a dog.'

Larry 'Curly' Haubner

When American Larry 'Curly' Haubner was asked for the secret to living 108 years, he flexed his biceps, flashed a mostly toothless smile and growled, 'Nutrition! Exercise!' In 2010, his 107th year, he was as vigorous as ever and at 5 feet 8 inches tall, weighed the same as when he enlisted in the Second World War, at 160 pounds. His blood pressure, blood sugar levels, kidney function, digestive process and muscle tinge were all tested regularly, and all were fine. He took no medication and he never got sick. He could lift his walker over his head and he lifted an eight kg lead ball at least 20 times a day. Larry was a self-proclaimed 'health nut', eating a plant-based wholefood diet rich in fruits, nuts and vegetables.

Salvatore Caruso

Salvatore Caruso was born on 2 November 1905, making him 108 years old in 2013. He had a stunning memory, remembering back 100 years to 1913 when his father died, and to when his mother and brother had nearly died during the great influenza pandemic of 1918–19. When asked how he had achieved his remarkable longevity, the centenarian said, 'No drinking, no smoking ... I have eaten mostly figs and beans while growing up and I have hardly ever eaten any red meat.'

Abdul Rahman Abu Bakar

Malaysia's oldest man, Abdul Rahman Abu Bakar or 'Pak Man', died of old age at his home in Kampung Denger, Bukit Puteri, in September 2012, age 117 (unconfirmed). Pak Man (as he liked to be called) attributed his longevity to, 'avoiding sweet, salty and milky foods, not smoking and eating lots and lots of local vegetables.' In over 100 years of life he never suffered diabetes, high blood pressure, stroke or heart disease of any sort. He read books without glasses and moved about without a walking stick.

Super-centenarian Magomed Labazanov

The elderly southern Russian, Magomed Labazanov, said he was born before the last tsar, Nicholas the Second, took the throne in 1890, although this is unconfirmed. Nevertheless, he was certainly a super-centenarian. His secrets were, 'abstaining from booze and tobacco ... and a diet high in fruits, corn, vegetables and wild garlic.'

Nina Johnson

The reason she's still alive in 2013? 'I didn't die,' she said. Johnson, aged 108, was born weighing less than two pounds and was not expected to survive.

Millia Dampier

Millia Dampier, aged 103 in 2013, still cooks breakfast, does her stretching exercises every morning 'to ward off stiffness', loves vegetables and enjoys 'running' up and down her front porch with her walker.

> If everyone felt as good as I did, there'd be no doctors!
>
> Irene Lavoie, 100, did not smoke or drink, and loves fruits and vegetables

Daisy Borrill

You've just got to love this woman. 'One of Britain's oldest women says the reason for her long life is her daily tonic – ogling pictures of burly men wearing nothing more than their underpants, on the calendar on her wall. 105-year-old Daisy Borrill says looking at physiques as impressive as David Beckham or Daniel Craig is what makes her life worth living. And the skimpier their trunks, the better. Daisy, who lives in a care home in Grimsby, Lincs, was delighted to receive a racy calendar for her recent birthday from her great-great niece Elaine Marsden. She says she's always been active and busy and has tried to live life to the full. Daisy acknowledges her calendars, saying that one of the men in her latest one is nearly nude. She says that she likes his little trunks. Daisy's favourite, according to Elaine, is Mr June, who is holding just a metal cylinder to cover his private parts.'[2]

Ed Ball Oberle

Ed turned 100 years old in June 2012. Ed has always been active, still drives and works out daily at San Jose Country Club. He said, 'I am in good condition for my age. I never in a million years ever thought I would be as old as this. I feel 39.'

Mildred Hays

100-year-old Mildred Hays was widowed in her mid-30s and then raised ten children. She had a passion for gardening (growing and eating her own fresh plants), walking (after Thanksgiving dinners she would take her family for a four-mile hike to the local reservoir and back, in her 70s and 80s), and learned to ride a bicycle at age 67.

Lois Williamson Morgan

Lois turned 100 in 2012.[3] Her family says, 'she lived a balanced life, had a positive attitude, was married to the love of her life, never smoked and exercised regularly.'

Jeralean Talley

As of July 2013, 114-year-old Jeralean Talley is the second oldest person alive. Jeralean is one of 11 siblings. She spent her younger years picking cotton and peanuts, and digging sweet potatoes. She says someone else is responsible for her long life and good humour. 'Don't ask me. Ask him,' she says, pointing to the sky. Talley did not drive but walked everywhere. She can still get around using a walker and gave up bowling at age 104, but she still plans to attend annual fishing outings.

> We walked to work and again at lunchtime. We always
> did a lot of walking. And ate wholesome foods.
>
> New Zealand twins, Alison Hunt and Audrey Duthie, age 100[4]

> Walk, grow your own vegetables,
> don't overeat and eat well-balanced meals.
>
> Magdalena Lee Skiff, 108

Queenie Kent and Nan

Queenie Kent, from Leichardt, turned 103 in 2010. She takes a brisk walk for 45 minutes every day to keep fit. She has been to hospital three times in 103 years. She has amazing vision, requires no walking or hearing aids and has never suffered from serious disease.

Nan (a friend of my mum's) is 94 years-old, slim as a rake and eats sparingly. She tends a stunning garden, grows her own vegetables, drives, and follows cricket and the horses. Her first-ever visit to a doctor was in 2008, at age 89, for a check-up. The doctor was staggered – there was absolutely nothing wrong with her!

The world's oldest doctor

Dr Shigeaki Hinohara, 100 years old, is Japan's guru of healthy aging. He eats just 1300 calories per day, about a third of the 3500 calorie average eaten by people in the Western world. How is he doing? Very well thanks.

Eat light and walk, walk, walk ...

American Verona Johnston, 114 years old, had a daily snack of freshly squeezed orange juice, one cracker, one cinnamon drop and one cashew. 'That's enough,' she insisted. Well into her 90s she continued to climb seven flights of stairs daily to stay in shape.

Nobel Prize winner Rita Levi-Montalcini, an Italian author of research on brain cells, hit 100 in 2009. She rises at 5 a.m. every day and eats once a day, at lunchtime. She says, 'I might allow myself a bowl of soup or an orange in the evening, but that's about it. I have never been ill ... my brain functions better today than it did when I was 20.'

At 102, Garnett Beckman doesn't want to be defined for her longevity as a centenarian, but as a little old lady who walks. She hiked the Grand Canyon each year from ages 75 to 91.

The 1800s to the 2010s

Henry Allington, aged 113, was once the world's oldest man. He lived a life that spanned three centuries: the 1800s, 1900s and 2000s.

American Lucille Salter was 104 years old in 2009. She recommends eating well and refraining from smoking and drinking to live a long life.

American Sam Abate turned 100 in September 2009 and retained a sharp mind and a great sense of humor. He suffered no heart disease or diabetes. He read biographies, watched political television shows and cooked home-made meals. He attributed his longevity to low stress, saying, 'stress is a killer'. He watched what he ate, took daily exercise and refused to let even the Great Depression get to him.

Mary Hamilton Brown, at 104 years old, has a great attitude. She has never been ill, takes no prescription medications and always wears a smile on her face. She said, 'I appreciate electricity. Back in the day you had a kerosene lamp to see by. Now all you have to do is push a button. I appreciate washing machines. I used to build a fire under a big pot of water to wash clothes. It is also easier to just go buy rice in the store. I used to beat rice into mortar for us to eat. We had a garden with plenty of fresh vegetables. I tried smoking, but I didn't like it, and I am glad I didn't learn to like it. Be good and kind, and don't lie and don't steal, and be honest and you will live long. And if you know better than to do something, don't do it.'

> Choose the right spouse; encourage sex –
> with your spouse that is …
> Dr Ephraim Engleman,100-years-old

Don't smoke, don't drink

Margaret Dell, at 96 years old, was the designated driver for her 70-year-old friends. She lived on the second floor of her building and was forced to walk up and down the stairs each day. She ate half a sandwich for lunch and had the rest for dinner, after her game of tennis. She never drank or smoked.

Lyster Holland, 101 years old in 2008, had 19 grandchildren and 33 great-grandchildren. He never smoked and rarely drank alcohol. 'I've had a good life, had a lot of experiences.'

American Camilla Svec turned 102 years old in 2009. She had clear eyes, a clear mind and a youthful spirit. She said, 'You know, I don't feel old. I have no serious illnesses. There are so many things I can still do.'

Bob Straight is 100 and still trim. He regularly exercises on a treadmill and bike, and when asked his secret he says, 'I never smoked nor drank, I didn't want to die.'[5]

Eva Curtis of Alton turned 101 years old on 3 February 2010. She outlived most of her family. Did she get her genes from her family? 'No,' she said, 'I eat right, I didn't smoke or drink.'

The world's oldest family

As of March 2010, the Hurlburt siblings were three brothers and five sisters ranging in age from 79 to 96 years old. Each is healthy, active and creative, and enjoys a good joke. 'Why did we live so long? It wasn't from overeating – there were 11 in our family.' They remember having soup for supper to stretch the food. Their longevity is not genetic, as their parents died at ages 45 and 63.[6]

Gladys Reynolds, 104 years old in January 2010, moves like a woman half her age with the grace of a ballet dancer. She has no family doctor, never smoked or drank, and takes no pills. She still drives her 1992 Lincoln.[7]

The world's oldest man ever?

Indian Habib Miyan died on 18 August 2008 at a reported 138 years old (this is unconfirmed). He was listed as the country's oldest man in India's *Limca Book of Records*. Without a birth certificate giving formal proof of his age, Habib (who played the clarinet in a maharaja's band before retiring in 1938) could not prove his longevity. His pension book showed his birth date as 20 May 1879, which would make him 129 years old at the very least. This makes him the oldest person ever recorded alive. When asked about the secret of his long life, he said, 'If you treat your body well, the body will treat you well.'

An active lifestyle

Japanese Yuichiro Miura became the first person ever to ski Mount Everest in 1970. Then in 2003, at age 70, he climbed it again, making him the oldest person ever to reach the roof of the world. Then he repeated it at age 75, and then he repeated it again, climbing to the top of the world's highest mountain at age 80, in 2013.[8] He ate hand-rolled sushi and drank green tea while up there.

American Frank Shearer first put on wooden plank water skis in 1939. In 2008, at 102 years old, Frank was in far better shape, and still kicking up the spray near his home in Washington state, US. 'I like the outdoors and the exercise,' he said.

> I've always eaten healthy food; I've never smoked and rarely drunk alcohol. The most important thing is laughter and a sense of humour.
>
> Ellen Watson, age 110

Lester Hazer

In a hilarious interview, Lester was asked, 'How many children did you have?' Lester said, 'I didn't have any, my wife had them. I would have had a hell of a time having them.' He was then asked, 'What do you do around here?' Lester said, 'Not any more than I have to. Well, I would say work; you're getting exercise every day you ain't sitting around drinking.' Lester was 100 at the time he was interviewed.

Sprinting and long-distance marathons

Japanese Kozo Haraguchi broke the 100-metre sprint record (for age group 95–99) in 2005, running it in 22.04 seconds at the age of 95! American Frank Ruebl, 90 years old in 2009, runs marathons.

Non-smoking, non-drinking vegetarian Fauja Singh ran his first marathon at age 89. He was part of the world's oldest marathon team called 'Sikhs in the City'. Fauja is now 101 years old, still running, still breaking world records and still recommends 'smiling'.

Hryhoriy Nestor died on 14 December 2007 at age 116. He credited his longevity to 'potatoes, exercise and healthy outdoor living'.

Yoga, pole vaulting and karate

Fumiyasu Yamakawa, age 86, trains daily, including his yoga practice, to prepare for an annual decathlon. His favourite events are high jump and pole vault.

Rosemary Braithwaite, 72 years old, is the oldest woman in New Zealand to earn her karate black belt.

Charlotte Forte received more than 100 birthday cards for her 100th birthday on 22 October 2009. Forte attributes her long life to nutrition. 'I think mainly, it's because of my information on health and that was at an early age. People at that time didn't know much about food. I had a lot of information that people didn't ordinarily know; I think I applied it in my life without even realising it. It makes you aware of what's in the food and what it does for you.'

Lew Hollander from Oregon became the second 80-year-old to complete the very challenging Ford Ironman World Championship in Kona, Hawaii. The event includes a 2.4-mile swim, a 112-mile bike ride and a 26.2-mile marathon run.

My secrets of longevity are simple: I stay positive, I contribute, I eat a healthy diet, and every morning I do yoga.

Teresa Hsu, age 113

It's not, 'the older you get, the sicker you get.' It's, 'the older you get, the healthier you've been.' The advantage of living to 100 is ... how you got there.

Dr Thomas Perls, Longevity Expert, who led The Centenarian Study

Chew your food, play music and don't take any medicines.

Ray DeLaurentis, age 101

I grew my own vegetables, I always had silverbeet.

Peg Griffin, moving into a rest home, age 107

Good health! That's about it. What else could I wish for? A few cents in the pocketbook doesn't mean that much if you don't feel good.

Rose Sprechman, age 105[9]

I don't drink. I've never smoked. I'm just glad to be in as good health as I am. I would be miserable if I were in the shape that others are in at this age. I've been taking Spanish lessons; I love to play bingo and the Wii, and I'm a crossword addict. Right now, when I go to the doctor, they can't find anything wrong with me. You've got to take care of yourself healthwise.

Lynn 'Mac' McMillan, age 100 and the retirement home-resident gardener

Morning exercise, I eat garlic and salads every day and have fish on Fridays.

Ozzie Pualte, age 100

Don't forget your greens.

Lillian Nana Irby, age 110

Eating when hungry, drinking when dry, sleeping when tired, and not letting other people tell me how to live.

Whalen Stensby, age 100

To lower fat content – reduce obesity – one must reduce calories taken in, or increase the output by increasing activity, or both. Eat a lower-calorie diet. Eat as little as you can get away with, and try to exercise more.

Dr Jules Hirsch, Emeritus Professor and Emeritus Physician-in-Chief at Rockefeller University, researcher of obesity for nearly 60 years[10]

If I had known I would live this long, I would have taken better care of myself.

Eubie Blake, jazz composer

Analysis of gene expression patterns by a molecular technique called 'microarray analysis' has shown that aging, calorically restricted mice show gene expression patterns resembling those of young animals. Calorie restriction also lowers cellular oxidative damage by reducing mitochondrial oxygen free radical production, lessens age-related telomere shortening, lowers inflammation, increases DNA damage repair efficiency and lowers damage to DNA and RNA (thus promoting genomic stability), lowers insulin levels while promoting insulin sensitivity, reduces the number of senescent (non-dividing) cells that accumulate with aging, attenuates age-related cellular protein cross-linking, and increases the removal of damaged cellular proteins, a process called 'autophagy', which declines with age and plays a role in resistance to infection, cancer, heart disease, and neurodegeneration.

Dr Sharon Hirsch, Pathology Resident, Tulane Medical Center, and Dr Rodney Shackelford, DO, PhD, Assistant Professor of Clinical Pathology, Tulane Medical Center, USA

I give credit to my longevity to one thing. Back then we lived off basics; good, basic food. There was no such thing as fast food.

Roy Raborn, 100 years old, 2013

What is the secret to long life? Clean living. Clean conscience. I like people. I love people.

Chick Pelonero, 100 years old, *The Chronicle Augusta*, 25 September 2013

I just turned 100 and I don't feel bad. I've been healthy. I never drank or smoked.

Beula Klopolsky, *The Reporter Herald*, 27 September 2013

Appendix B
Juice recipes

To make the juices

Cut up and feed ingredients through your juice extractor to make a power-packed vegetable juice blend. Sip on this while fasting, or drink three times a day while fasting. Double or halve the recipe where required.

SuperGreen Detoxer

10 or so leaves spinach,
    kale or silverbeet
2–3 sticks celery
1 cucumber
1 carrot
1 peeled lemon
handful of fresh parsley

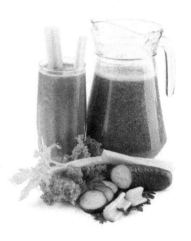

You can't get much greener than this and still have it taste delicious! Full of essential nutrients and great for every system of the body.

FastMaster Special

4 sticks celery
2 carrots
1 medium beetroot
1 peeled lemon

1 large, peeled knob of ginger
(equivalent to 1 teaspoon)
handful of fresh parsley

This is one of our favourite basic fasting blends. It has a range of flavours and if you're a few days into your fast, you can taste every single drop of goodness. Great to have stored as a staple in the fridge while fasting.

Beetroot Zinger

5 cm piece of ginger, peeled
2 celery sticks
1 beetroot

1 green apple
½ cucumber

Beetroot juice is a winning ingredient in any juice fast. Mix with apple, celery, cucumber and ginger to create a delicious, heart-healthy, healing drink.

Classic Carrot

6–8 carrots
1 large, peeled knob of ginger
  (equivalent to 1 teaspoon)
1 peeled lemon (optional)

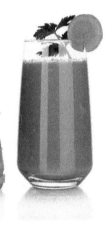

The classic carrot is a great juice if you're feeling low in energy during a fast and need an instant sugar hit. This one is particularly good during those low slumps in the afternoon or first thing in the morning. It's hard to beat the carotene-filled Classic Carrot!

Clean Green Special

6 sticks celery
1 large, peeled knob of ginger
  (equivalent to 1 teaspoon)
1 peeled lemon
½ cucumber

½ head of broccoli
½ green apple (optional)
handful of kale
handful of mint

If you're looking for a really refreshing, green cleansing juice, then this one is for you! Full of essential nutrients and wonderfully cleansing, this is great on a hot summer afternoon enjoyed in the sunshine.

The Unique Kiwi

1 beetroot
2 carrots
3 medium kumara/sweet potato
  (or ¼ pumpkin)

1 large, peeled knob of ginger
  (equivalent to 1 teaspoon
  – optional)

This juice is something special. The delicious New Zealand kumara gives it a creamy texture and the beetroot and carrot enhance its sweetness.

Grapefruit Chill

1 grapefruit
1 cucumber
½ cup of mint leaves

Grapefruit is bursting with living enzymatic activity and is packed with vitamins and antioxidants; and it naturally burns fat! Have this juice first thing on your fasting morning to waken your taste buds and digestive system. On a summer's day, freeze into ice cubes for a refreshing fasting treat.

Bowel Soother

3 dandelion leaves
1 cup cabbage leaves
1 green apple (with skin)

2.5 cm peeled ginger
½ cucumber
handful of fresh mint leaves

Anyone experiencing constipation, gas or bloating will benefit from drinking this juice. Cabbage leaves are particularly calming and soothing for your bowels.

Liver Lover

3 dandelion leaves
2 carrots
2.5 cm peeled ginger
1 clove garlic
½ cup broccoli pieces

handful of fresh parsley
handful of rocket leaves
turmeric or dandelion root
(if you can find it – optional)

This juice packs a powerful punch. It is rich in liver-nourishing nutrients, and the strong, bitter flavour will also stimulate bile flow, creating a powerful cleansing effect. Be warned, it will stimulate your taste buds!

Recipe contributors: Tracey Bennett, Andrea Frires, Jules Recordon, Nicky Utting

Notes

AIM	*Archives of Internal Medicine*
AFP	Agence France-Presse
AASLD	American Association for the Study of Liver Diseases
AICR	American Institute for Cancer Research
AP	Associated Press
ARIC	Atherosclerosis Risk in Communities
BMC	*BioMed Central (BMC)*
BMI	body mass index
BMJ	*British Medical Journal*
BWH	Brigham and Women's Hospital
CNIO	Spanish National Cancer Research Centre
DHA	Dubai Health Authority
ECDC	European Centre for Disease Prevention and Control
EPIC	European Prospective Investigation into Cancer and Nutrition
GBD	Global Burden of Disease Study
GDA	*Growth, Development and Aging*
HSPH	Harvard School of Public Health
IARC	International Agency for Research on Cancer
IHME	The Institute for Health Metrics and Evaluation
ILC-UK	International Longevity Centre
JACC	*The Journal of the American College of Cardiology*
JAMA	*The Journal of the American Medical Association*
MESA	Multi-Ethnic Study of Atherosclerosis
MUSC	Medical University of South Carolina
NCDs	non-communicable diseases
NHANES	National Health and Nutrition Examination Surveys
NHS	National Health Service
NIH	National Institute of Health
OECD	Organisation for Economic Co-operation and Development
OCS	Okinawa Centenarian Study
PHP	Practitioner Health Program
TIFR	Tata Institute of Fundamental Research
UICC	Union for International Cancer Control
UKIOM	UK Institute of Medicine
USA	United States of America
USDA HNRCA	USDA Human Nutrition Research Center on Aging
WCRF	World Cancer Research Fund
WHO	World Health Organisation
YHA	Yemeni Heart Association

1. I know what it is like to be sick, really sick

1. 'The Longevity Risk and Reward for Middle-Income Americans' surveyed 500 Americans aged 55 to 75 and found that declining health is the number one concern for middle-income Americans. Survey by the Bankers Life and Casualty Company Center for a Secure Retirement. Reported by PRNewswire, 2 April 2013.

2. 'There is concern, and a lot of literature to support it, that there will be a generation of children who will die before their parents. They will be so fat that they will develop diabetes, cancer, heart disease – there's an endless list.' From Cardiff and Vale University Health Board statistics. Reported by walesonline.co.uk, 15 January 2012.

3. Norm R.C. Campbell, MD, from the University of Calgary in Alberta, and colleagues. 'As a result, it is predicted the next generation will live a shorter life span. If this occurs, it will be the first decline in life span since industrialization.' *The Canadian Journal of Cardiology* (online edition), 2012.

4. Study released by the Paris-based Organisation for Economic Co-operation and Development (OECD), 21 February 2012.

5. This economic longevity research study by The Institute for Health Metrics and Evaluation (IHME), was released to health reporters and researchers at the Association of Health Care Journalists Atlanta conference on 18 April 2012.

6. Study released by the British Heart Foundation and the University of Oxford. *The Daily Mail*, 12 August 2013.

2. Non-communicable diseases: a global crisis?

1. A study confirmed that there are now nearly one in nine adults, or 500,000,000 people, clinically obese, and more than one in ten of the world's adult population is now overweight. The study was published in *The Lancet*, 17 May 2013 and reported by Deutsche Welle, 18 May 2013.

2. *Ibid.*

3. The international developed countries' weight list as compiled by the Bloomberg news service using data from the Word Health Organisation (WHO), the Organisation for Economic Co-operation and Development (OECD) and a survey funded by the United States Agency for International Development. As reported by the *New Zealand Herald* (*NZ Herald*), 24 May 2013. Also see 'Obesity: preventing and managing the global epidemic', WHO, Geneva, 1998.

4. Three studies analysed together, covering the overall global levels of obesity, cholesterol and blood pressure and published in *The Lancet*, 2012. Also see The Council of Australian Government's Reform report on the National Healthcare Agreement, 24 May 2013.

5. Study by Sarah C. Walpole, David Prieto-Merino, Phil Edwards, John Cleland, Gretchen Stevens and Ian Roberts, 'The weight of nations: an estimation of adult human biomass'. *BMC Public Health*, 17 June 2012. Also see studies published in *The Lancet*, 4 February 2012.

6. Two billion people worldwide will be overweight by 2015, and more than 700 million will be obese, according to an EU-funded research study by North Carolina University nutrition lecturer Professor Barry Popkin, who examined exercise and working habits across the EU. Reported by news.wbfo.org, 17 October 2013.

7. Study by C.J. Murray and A.D. Lopez, Harvard School of Public Health, Boston, Massachusetts, USA. *The Lancet*, 24 May 1997, 349 (9064):1498–504.

8. Study from the near-decade long 'Early Childhood Longitudinal Study' by researchers on nearly 6000 white, black and Hispanic children. *Pediatrics*, December 2011.

9. From an International Diabetes Federation report released at the European Association for the Study of Diabetes congress in Lisbon, Portugal, 13–14 September 2011.

10. According to the Centers for Disease Control and Prevention (CDC), in 1980, 2% of adult-onset diabetes cases were diagnosed in people under the age of 19. In 2000 it was close to 50%.

11. A. Green, A.K. Sjølie, O. Eschøj, and K. Cruickshank, 'Epidemiology of diabetes mellitus' in J.C. Pickup and G. Williams (eds), *Textbook of Diabetes*, 2nd edition, Oxford, Blackwell Science, 1997. Also two studies by the University of California at San Francisco, Columbia University and researchers from the Institute for Preventive Medicine in Copenhagen, who analysed data on 276,835 people, who had been first examined in 1930. *New England Journal of Medicine*, 2010.

12. Study released by the OECD, 21 February 2012. Also see N.A. Roper, R.W. Bilous, W.F. Kelly, N.C. Unwin, and V.M. Connolly, 'Excess mortality in a population with diabetes and the impact of material deprivation: longitudinal population based study.' *British Medical Journal* (*BMJ*), 2001, 322:1389–93.

13. Obesity now outnumbers hunger worldwide according to an annual World Disasters Report released by the International Federation of the Red Cross, 22 September 2011.

14. *The 2013 Burden of Disease Study*, as released by the Ministry of Health and University of Otago researchers, 8 August 2013.

15. A quarter of New Zealand adults are now obese, one of the highest rates in the West and an increase of 150% since 1980. 'Number of obese or overweight Kiwi children to hit 25%'. Reported by the *Press*, 25 September 2010, and The 2006/2007 New Zealand Health Survey.

16. South Auckland obesity rates reported on 24 April 2013 by the *NZ Herald*. Also see a study released by the New Zealand Ministry of Health, 'A focus on nutrition, key findings of the 2008/2009 New Zealand adult nutrition survey' by the University of Otago.

17. The 2006/2007 New Zealand Health Survey. Also see note 42.

18. From the 2011 State of the Nation Report from market researcher Roy Morgan Research.

19. Health Ministry data as released to the *Press*, published 25 September 2010.

20. A 2010 Ministry of Health report, 'Diabetes Policy Model', reveals that 10% of the adult population will have type II diabetes by 2028 and nearly half a million people by 2036. Diabetes New Zealand National President, Chris Baty, said that number was conservative as cases were already higher than projections and increasing by 8% a year.

21. In New Zealand, the lifetime risk of developing bowel cancer is 1 in 18 for men and 1 in 23 for women. 'Nutrition and the Burden of Disease: New Zealand 1997–2011', The Ministry of Health and The University of Auckland 2003. Also see National Cancer Registry (2008); District Health Board (DHB) http://www.bowelscreeningwaitemata.co.nz/BowelHealth/BowelcancerinNZ.aspx; http://www.bowelcheck.co.nz/; www.bowelcanceraustralia.org/bca/, 2010.

22. Study by University of Otago researchers Dr Kirsten Coppell and Professor Jim Mann and colleagues, from the University's Edgar National Centre for Diabetes and Obesity Research. *New Zealand Medical Journal*, 1 March 2013.

23. See note 3.

24. Study published in *Obesity*, January 2011. The study claimed that by 2025 the number of obese Australians will surpass those of healthy weight.

25. The Council of Australian Governments (COAG) Reform released their fourth report on the National Healthcare Agreement on 24 May 2013. Also see study by the Australian Institute of Health and Welfare (AIHW), January 2012. The researchers found that since 1990 the prevalence of diabetes in the Australian population has nearly tripled, from 1.5% to 4.1%.

26. 'Comparative Health Performance in the Asia-Pacific Region: Findings and Implications of the Global Burden of Disease Study 2010.' Released by IHME at their Australian conference in Melbourne, 2–3 May 2013.

27. 'Action Agenda 2013.' A report from Obesity Australia that is a five-point Action Agenda taking in research from the International Obesity Summit in New Zealand, December 2012.

28. The survey by the Centre for Community Child Health at Royal Children's Hospital in Melbourne, and Adelaide researchers, as collected from 4983 preschoolers aged four and five in 2004, showed more than 15% were overweight and a further 5.5% now met the clinical definition of obese.

29. *Medical Journal of Australia*, 20 February 2012.

30. The Wellness Index, by Roy Morgan Research. A survey of 50,000 Australians, 16 April 2013.

31. The Australian Bureau of Statistics' (ABS) quarterly snapshot of society, released 10 December 2009.

32. A landmark study of more than 16,000 Australians that used results from the Australian National Health Survey 2004–2005, which were analysed by the University of Sydney and Deakin International. *Journal of Obesity*, 2010.

33. Reported in the *Australian and New Zealand Journal of Public Health*, January 2009. Also see The Australian National Children's Nutrition and Physical Activity Survey, jointly funded by the Department of Health and Ageing, the Department of Agriculture, Fisheries and Forestry and the Australian Food and Grocery Council, October 2008.

34. Indian obesity and diabetes statistics from the 2013 OECD study as reported by United Nations News on 16 April 2013. Also The RV Metropolis Bangalore Survey (April 2012–June 2013) found that type II diabetes is increasing in the 20–29 age group.

35. *Ibid.*

36. Indian obesity and diabetes statistics from the 2013 OECD study in note 34. Also, India has 20% adult obesity rates in 2011, from a study conducted among urban Indian adolescents by the National Diabetes, Obesity and Cholesterol Foundation.

37. Chinese obesity rates reported by *China Daily*, 30 May 2013.

38. Summary released 9 January 2012 by The Chinese Health Education Center.

39. See note 37.

40. Study paper published in *The Lancet*, 2012. In 30 years, the Chinese people have gone from having barely enough to eat to almost 100 million diabetics, with diabetes now afflicting nearly 10% of Chinese adults.

41. Reported by market research firm QF Information Consulting, 8 December 2011. Also see a 2009 report by the Chinese Association for Student Nutrition and Health. The number of overweight young people aged between 7 and 17 had tripled between 1982 and 2002.

42. Three studies covering the overall global levels of obesity, cholesterol and blood pressure, as published in *The Lancet*, 2012, show that over 10% of the global population is now obese, doubling that of 1980 – just 30 years ago.

43. Study published in the *New England Journal of Medicine*, March 2010, found much higher rates of diabetes than previous studies.

44. Ryan K. Masters, PhD, 'The Impact of Obesity on US Mortality Levels: The Importance of Age and Cohort Factors in Population Estimates.' Masters is a Robert Wood Johnson Foundation Health and Society Scholar and Demographer at Columbia University's Mailman School of Public Health in New York City, and Associate Professor of Sociology at the University of Colorado, Boulder, USA. *American Journal of Health*, 5 April 2013.

45. Obesity predictions in the USA released by the Trust for America's Health and the Robert Wood Johnson Foundation in January 2012. Also see a study published in the *American Journal of Preventive Medicine*, 2012, that found that by 2030, 42% of US adults could be obese.

46. Published in *Obesity*, the research is based on the US government's Agency for Healthcare Research and Quality, government survey data collected between the 1970s and 2004, suggesting that 86% of American adults will be overweight by 2030, with an obesity rate of 51%.

47. See note 3.

48. See note 42.

49. Study by researchers from Northwestern University as reported at the 2011 Scientific Sessions of the American Heart Association, finding 83% of US men and 72% of US women will be overweight or obese by the year 2020.

50. Study by Franco Sassi, the OECD Senior Health Economist and former London School of Economics lecturer, who worked on the report for three years. September, 2010.

51. According to the SEARCH for Diabetes in Youth Population Study, sponsored by the CDC and National Institute of Health (NIH), and data published by the Institute of Medicine (IOM) in 2006, obesity rates for preschool children and adolescents have more than tripled in the past 30 years.

52. The 2013 Ministry of Health Report was presented at Otago University's Waistline seminar on 7 June 2013. Also see D.E. King *et al.*, 'The status of baby boomers' health in the US: The healthiest generation?' *Journal of American Medical Association*, 2013, DOI:10.1001/jamainternmed.2013.2006.

53. 2011 diabetes statistics released by the CDC.

54. *Ibid.* If Americans keep living a sedentary lifestyle, filled with junk food and starch, a third will be diabetic by the year 2050.

55. New York obesity rates reported by the *New York Daily News* and Agence France-Presse (AFP), 10 June 2013.

56. American Samoa childhood obesity rates data from the Alpert Medical School at Brown University. Study of 800 babies born in American Samoa between 2001 and 2008.

57. Report published in the *Canadian Journal of Public Health*, 2013, covering the period from 2003–2011, showed self-reported adult obesity rates in Canada have increased to 25%.

58. See note 3.
59. Study published in *Diabetologia, the Journal of the European Association for the Study of Diabetes*, June 2013. The study covered patient records in both Britain and Canada. Also see figures from the Women's College Research Institute in Toronto, Canada, and Sahlgrenska Academy at the University of Gothenburg in Sweden.
60. See note 58.
61. Study released 10 April 2012 by Brazil's Health Ministry, based on up-to-date data on 54,144 people in the capital of Brazil's 27 states.
62. Mexico obesity and diabetes rates released by Mexico's 2012 Secretariat of Health. President Felipe Calderon said that 'Mexico had the highest rate of obesity for children ages 5 to 19 in the world.' Reported by Associated Press (AP) and the *Washington Post*, 20 October 2011.
63. European obesity rates reported by Deutsche Welle, 18 May 2013. Also see *Health at a Glance: Europe 2010*, a report on health in the 27-member bloc by the OECD and the Brussels-based Commission. The report confirmed the rate of obesity has more than doubled over the past 20 years in most member states.
64. *Ibid*.
65. European obesity rates reported by Deutsche Welle, 18 May 2013.
66. German obesity and diabetes rates taken from a 2012 Government Report. Reported by Deutsche Welle, 17 December 2012.
67. See note 65.
68. Turkish obesity rates released by the Turkish Statistics Institute (TurkStat). Reported by worldbulletin.net, 25 April 2013.
69. The British National Child Measurement Programme, 2011, found that one child in three is overweight when they leave primary school at the age of 11. Almost a fifth are classed as obese. Also, according to 2011 figures gathered by the National Health Service (NHS), the number of final year primary school children classed as obese has risen to 19%.
70. The NHS 2011 Survey, reported by Top News, 14 December 2011.
71. UK diabetes and obesity rates in young people study by researchers from Cardiff University and the Heart of England NHS Trust in Birmingham. *Diabetes, Obesity and Metabolism*, June 2013.
72. According to a European Commission report published in November 2011, the UK is the most overweight and obese country in Europe. Reported on 11 March 2012 by independent.com.
73. UK obesity and diabetes rates reported by the *Daily Record*, 21 June 2013.
74. High blood pressure and obesity death numbers from the 2010 GBD study published in *The Lancet*. Also, the 2010 Heart and Stroke Statistics report published by the American Heart Association, WHO and an international consortium of nearly 500 scientists from 187 countries globally, including the Harvard School of Public Health.
75. British diabetes rates and medication sales reported by NHS data from the Health and Social Care Information Centre for England, show Britain's diabetes prescriptions soared by 50% in six years. Reported by *The Daily Mail*, 14 August 2012.
76. World obesity rates, *The Lancet*, 17 May 2013. Reported by Deutsche Welle, 18 May 2013.
77. The Scottish obesity crisis is worse than previously thought as the Scottish Government had published the wrong figures. Corrected numbers were released by the Scottish Government and the Scottish Health Survey on 2 August 2013.
78. *Ibid*.
79. Reported by Diet Chef and PRNewswire from Edinburgh, Scotland on 8 October 2012.
80. Scottish children and obesity rates data from a study covering 52,139 children, 'weighed and measured' children of primary one age, reported by BBC News, 30 April 2013.
81. Irish childhood obesity rates from The Framework for Preventing and Addressing Overweight and Obesity in Northern Ireland 2012–2022: 'A Fitter Future for All.' Reported by *The Independent*, 15 April 2013.
82. E.L. Masso, S. Gonzalez, S. Johansson, MA, L.A. Garcia Rodriguez, 'Trends in the prevalence and incidence of diabetes in the UK: 1996–2005'. *Journal of Epidemiology and Community Health*, 2009.
83. 2013 statistics as reported by the NHS Health and Social Care Information Centre (HSCIC).
84. Study led by Dr Sonia Saxena of Imperial College London and researchers from the Medical

University of South Carolina and the Imperial School of Public Health, with data from the National Health Service UK health statistics. PLoS ONE, 13 June 2013.

85. UK obesity rates. Reported by *The Telegraph* and agencies, 29 October 2012.

86. A study conducted by researchers from the University College London showed the number of children in the UK taking prescription weight-loss drugs increased by 15 times between 1999 and 2006. *British Journal of Clinical Pharmacology*, reported by the *Observer*, 25 October 2009.

87. French obesity rates, *The Telegraph*, 16 October 2012. Also see note 42.

88. *ibid.*

89. *ibid.*

90. Middle East obesity and diabetes statistics released by Mohammed Al Kebsi, Consultant Interventional Cardiologist from the Yemeni Heart Association (YHA), at the first International Cardiology Symposium and Diabetes Forum – A Global Agenda (ICS-13), May 2013.

91. *ibid.*

92. 'Over 80% of Kuwait children are obese,' said Professor Mustafa Hayat at the Basic Education Faculty, 17 December 2012. Reported by *alshahed Daily*.

93. Study conducted among 230,000 adolescents by Israel Clalit Health Services reveals that 1 in 11 teenagers in Israel suffer from severe obesity. Also, according to 2011 Health Ministry surveys, about half of the country's population is overweight.

94. See note 75.

95. Statistics taken from a Dubai Health Authority (DHA) campaign linked to World Heart Day, 29 September 2011.

96. Study published in the *Journal of Paediatrics and Child Health*, late 2011.

97. Belly fat and heart death risk. Study by S. Adabag, *et al.*, 'Risk of sudden cardiac death in obese individuals: The Atherosclerosis Risk in Communities (ARIC) study'. Presented by the Heart Rhythm Society 2012, abstract PO1-67.

98. 'Heart Disease and Stroke Statistics – 2012 Update' is a study published online in *Circulation: Journal of the American Heart Association*, 15 December 2011.

99. US heart failure predictions study analysis published in *Circulation: Heart Failure*, 24 April 2013.

100. 'Older Americans 2010: Key Indicators of Well-Being', a report compiled by 15 federal agencies in July 2010. The report found that the rate of death from Alzheimer's rose almost 30-fold, from 6 per 100,000 people in 1981 to 176.9 per 100,000 in 2006.

101. B. Jarett *et al.*, 'Lifetime Risks of Cardiovascular Disease.' *The New England Journal of Medicine*, 2012.

102. See note 75.

103. WHO estimates that the number of people that will die from cardiovascular diseases each year will reach 23.3 million by 2030.

104. Report from the National Center for Cardiovascular China confirmed that China has 290 million patients with cardiovascular disease, 60 million more than the 230 million such patients in 2010. Reported by mizonews.com, 9 August 2013.

105. See note 21.

106. The Australian Bureau of Statistics, August 2013.

107. Indian heart disease numbers shared by Dr Khawar Kazmi, Section Head of Cardiology at Aga Khan University Hospital, during a talk on 2012 World Heart Day.

108. *ibid.*

109. *ibid.*

110. Senior Cardiologist and Secretary of the Pakistan Cardiology Society, Professor Khan Shahzaman, said at a seminar on 29 September 2011, 'By 2020 non-communicable diseases (NCDs) would account for 73% of Pakistani deaths, of which 50% would be cardiovascular disease.'

111. See note 107.

112. *ibid.*

113. Heart disease mortality expectations study on data from five long-running studies of US heart health, 1964–2008, published in *The Journal of the American Medical Association* (*JAMA*) by Northwestern University cardiologist John Wilkins and colleagues, 7 November 2012. Also see a US heart disease mortality study by Brent M. Egan, MD, Professor of Medicine and Pharmacology at Medical University of South Carolina (MUSC), and colleagues, published in *Circulation*, 2013. The research

was analysed using National Health and Nutrition Examination Surveys (NHANES) from three key study periods: 1988–1994, 1999–2004 and 2005–2010; reported 2 July 2013.

114. *ibid.*
115. *ibid.*
116. *ibid.*
117. Study by B. Jarett *et al.*, 'Lifetime Risks of Cardiovascular Disease.' *The New England Journal of Medicine*, 27 January 2012.
118. See note 113.
119. W. Ashton, K. Nanchahal and D. Wood, 'Body mass index and metabolic risk factors for coronary heart disease in women.' *European Heart Journal*, 2001, 22: 46–55. Also see European Cardiovascular Disease Statistics provided by the European Heart Network and the European Society of Cardiology, 2013.
120. 'Cancer Facts & Figures 2010', an annual publication of the American Cancer Society in Atlanta, Georgia. Also see cancer report by the Union for International Cancer Control (UICC) and the International Agency for Research on Cancer (IARC), released on World Cancer Day, 4 February 2013.
121. 'Global Cancer Facts & Figures 2008' from an American Cancer Society news release, 4 February 2011.
122. *ibid.*
123. *ibid.*
124. University of Washington researchers, led by co-author Dr Rafael Lozano, a Professor of Global Health at the university's IHME, collected data from more than 300 cancer registries and cause-of-death offices in 187 countries. *The Lancet*, online edition, 15 September 2001.
125. The UK obesity and cancer connection figures from Cancer Research UK and World Cancer Research Fund 2012, 3 October 2012. Also see note 121.
126. Stomach cancer growth figures supplied by The American Cancer Society and reported by WHO on 6 May 2013. Also see note 121.
127. Research released by the American Institute for Cancer Research (AICR), 5 November 2009. Also see note 121.
128. *Health at a Glance: Europe 2010.* A report on health in the 27-member bloc by the OECD.
129. 'The Global Tobacco Epidemic, 2011: Warning about the Dangers of Tobacco', WHO Report, Geneva, Switzerland, 2011. Also see 'How Tobacco Smoke Causes Disease – The Biology and Behavioral Basis for Smoking-Attributable Disease', US Department of Health and Human Service.
130. R. Peto, A. Lopez, J. Boreham, M. Thun and C.J. Heath, *Mortality from Smoking in Developed Countries, 1950–2000*, Oxford University Press, New York, 1994. Also see 'A review of human carcinogens. Part E: Personal habits and indoor combustions', International Agency for Research on Cancer (IARC) Working Group on the Evaluation of Carcinogenic Risks to Humans, Lyon, France, IARC, 2009.
131. Cancer numbers taken from the most comprehensive global examination ever done on cancer, *The World Cancer Report*, IARC. Also see 'Nutrition, Physical Activity and Non-Communicable Disease Prevention: A Briefing Document.' Also 'The International Update of Alcohol-Linked Cancer Deaths, 2013.'
132. *ibid.*
133. See notes 21 and 131.
134. *ibid.*
135. *ibid.*
136. Study published in *Pharmaceutical Research*, 2008. The researchers said, 'Only 5% to 10% of all cancer cases can be attributed to genetic defects, while the remaining 90% to 95% have their roots in the environment and lifestyle ... cancer is a disease commonly believed to be preventable.' Also see note 131.
137. Study published online, Obesity Reviews, 4 June 2012.
138. Chinese cancer growth figures from a report in *Chinese Medical Journal*, 13 June 2013.
139. See note 121.
140. The American Association for Cancer Research, *The 2013 Cancer Progress Report*. Reported by MedPage Today, 17 September 2013.

141. UK cancer numbers from the 2013 Macmillan Cancer Support Review, analysing existing data on cancer prevalence, incidence and mortality, 7 June 2013. Also see UK obesity and cancer connection figures from Cancer Research UK and World Cancer Research Fund, 2012.
142. UK breast cancer growth in young women, the *Guardian*, 3 May 2013.
143. See note 140.
144. The World Cancer Research Fund released figures on 4 February 2012 to mark World Cancer Day. They said, 'Ireland will have 35,500 new cancer cases a year by 2030.'

3. Advertising, marketing and medicine

1. Study by a research team from the University of Sydney and the Cancer Council NSW, *International Journal of Pediatric Obesity* (2010), May 2010.
2. *ibid.*
3. Reported by the *Sydney Morning Herald* and AAP, 29 April 2009.
4. Study by the Yale University's Rudd Center for Food Policy, 2009.
5. Elizabeth Russell interview and quotes reported by the *Sunday Star Times*, 2 May 2010.
6. Dr Pauline W. Chen, *New York Times*, 16 September 2010.
7. The 2010 GBD study published in *The Lancet*. Also see the 351-page World Cancer Report; Global Cancer Facts & Figures 2013; *Nutrition, Physical Activity and Non-Communicable Disease Prevention: A Briefing Document*; the Global Morbidity Report, 2008.
8. Study published in *Academic Medicine*, a journal of the Association of American Medical Colleges, 2010.
9. Study by S.N. Bleich *et al.*, 'Impact of physician BMI on obesity care and beliefs.' *Obesity 2012*, DOI: 10.1038/oby.2011.402, at the Johns Hopkins Bloomberg School of Public Health in Baltimore, reported by MedPage Today, 29 January 2012.
10. Nurses were more likely to be obese when compared to other professions. Study from the US Gallup-Healthways Well-Being Index poll of 138,438 people over 18 years old, 16 May 2013.
11. 'Invisible Patients', a government-funded 2009–10 study into the scale of the alcohol and drug abuse crisis in the British Medical Establishment. *Archives of Surgery*, 24 February 2012.
12. The Practitioner Health Program (PHP) was set up by the Chief Medical Officer for England, Sir Liam Donaldson, in response to concerns that health professionals were avoiding treatment for serious health problems and/or self-medicating, out of fear of being judged and stigmatised. Reported by Jane Dreaper, Health Correspondent, *BBC News*, 29 January 2010.
13. Study by T. D. Shanafelt *et al.*, 'Burnout and satisfaction with work-life balance among US physicians relative to the general US population.' *Archives of Internal Medicine*, 2012, 10.1001/archinternmed.2012.3199. Reported by MedPage Today, 20 August 2012.
14. Read more at http://www.sacbee.com/static/weblogs/run_sacramento/2010/04/80-year-old-boston-runnerdoctor-talks-longevity.html#ixzz0rdEjoDwe
15. See our website, www.jasonshonbennett.for many more references and further information concerning breast cancer.
16. 'Expert Report, Food, Nutrition, Physical Activity, and the Prevention of Cancer: a Global Perspective', Word Cancer Research Fund (WCRF) and AICR, 2007–11.
17. B. Starfield, 'Is US health really the best in the world?' *JAMA* 284, 2000, pp. 483–85.
18. D. Phillips, N, Christenfeld and L. Glynn, 'Increase in US medication-error death between 1983 and 1993', *The Lancet* 351, pp. 643–44.
19. R.N. Anderson, 'Deaths: leading causes for 2000.' National Vital Statistics Reports 50(16) (2002). *The Lancet* 351, 1998, pp. 643–44.
20. US Congressional House Subcommittee Oversight Investigation, 'Cost and quality of healthcare: unnecessary surgery', Washington DC, 1976. Also see L. Leape, 'Unnecessary surgery', *Annual Review of Public Health* 13, 1992, pp. 363–83.
21. J. Lazarou, B. Pomeranz, and P.N. Corey, 'Incidence of adverse drug reactions in hospitalized patients', *JAMA* 279, 1998, pp. 1200–05. Also see 'International Drug Monitoring: the Role of the Hospital', WHO Technical Report Series No. 425, Geneva, Switzerland, 1966.
22. A survey by the European Centre for Diseases Prevention and Control (ECDC) covering 1000

hospitals in 30 European countries, found a total of 15,000 reported healthcare-associated infections, meaning 1 in 18 patients in European hospitals had at least one hospital-acquired infection, leading to 3.2 million patients getting sick per year. Marc Sprenger, Director of the Stockholm-based ECDC said, 'Healthcare-associated infections pose a major public health problem and a threat to European patients.' Reported by Reuters Health Information, 5 July 2013.
23. Commentary article, *Nature*, 28 March 2012.

4. How do we get from where we are, to where we want to be?

1. C.L. Haynes and G.A. Cook, 'Audit of health promotion practice within a UK hospital: results of a pilot study'. *Journal of Evaluation in Clinical Practice*, 2008, 14:103–109.

5. Eat Less, Live Long

1. Study released at a International Longevity Centre UK (ILC-UK) event, 22 July 2013.
2. Research from the Pennington Biomedical Research Center in Louisiana, and Epworth's Centre for Molecular Biology and Medicine.
3. Study in *Journals of Gerontology Series A: Biological Sciences and Medical Sciences*, October 2007. Also see research by the UB School of Public Health and Health Professions and the University at Buffalo.
4. Research by the Salk Institute for Biological Studies in La Jolla, California in *Nature*.

6. Calorie restriction

1. Study by a team led by Maria Blasco, the Director of the Spanish National Cancer Research Centre (CNIO) and head of the Telomeres and Telomerase Group, Plos One, January 2013.
2. Study by Anderson *et al.*, *Circulation*, 2013.
3. Study by Honig, *et al.*, *Journal of the American Medical Association – Neurology*, 2012. 4. Also see a study by Phillips *et al.*, *Psychosomatic Medicine*, 2013.
5. R. Walford, chapter 5, pp. 51–73 in R. Kotulak and P. Gorer (eds), *Aging On Hold – Secrets of Living Younger Longer'*, Tribune Publishing, USA, (1992). Also see R.B. Effros, R.L. Walford, R. Weindruch and C.J. MitchELtree, 'Influences of dietary restriction on immunity to influenza in aged mice', *Gerontol*, July 1991, 46(4):B 142–147. Also a study by Chinese researchers from the Institute of Nutritional Sciences of the Chinese Academy of Sciences, reported in *China Daily*, 18 July 2013.
6. C. Sherwood, *et al.*, 'Aging of the cerebral cortex differs between humans and chimpanzees', *Proceedings of the National Academy of Sciences*, DOI:10.1073/pnas.1016709108, 25 July 2011, reported by Reuters, Columbus Public Health, Centers for Medicare and Medicaid Services, Centers for Disease Control and Prevention and NIH, 30 August 2012.
7. Professor Leonard Guarente, Donmez, Diana Wang, Dena E. Cohen, and Paul F. Glenn, 'SIRT1 Suppresses β-Amyloid Production by Activating the α-Secretase Gene ADAM10Gizem', the Laboratory and Department of Biology, Massachusetts Institute of Technology, Cambridge, MA 02139, USA, *Cell*, 23 July 2010. Also see Michael J. Powell, Mathew C. Casimiro, Carlos Cordon-Cardo, Xiaohong He, Wen-Shuz Yeow, Chenguang Wang, Peter McCue, Michael W McBurney and Richard G Pestell, 'Disruption of a Sirt1 Dependent Autophagy Checkpoint in the Prostate Results in Prostatic Intraepithelial Neoplasia Lesion Formation', *Cancer Research*, 1 February 2011. Also see 40 years of published medical literature covering European wartime populations and Okinawans, Washington University School of Medicine, *JAMA*, 2007; 297(9):986–94. See a study by Tomas A. Prolla, a UW-Madison Professor of Genetics, John M. Denu of UW-Madison's Wisconsin Institute for Discovery, postdoctoral fellows Shinichi Someya, of UW-Madison and the University of Tokyo, and Wei Yu of UW-Madison, *Cell*, November 2010.
8. *ibid.*
9. *ibid.* See also studies by researchers from the Tata Institute of Fundamental Research (TIFR), Department of Biological Sciences, *Cell* reports and *Molecular and Cellular Biology*, January 2013.
10. See notes 7 and 9.
11. *Nature*, 21 September 2011.
12. *Science*, 16 April 2010.

13. *ibid*; see additional notes and references on our website, www.jasonshonbennett.com.
14. Study presented by Dr Sebastiaan Hammer of Leiden (the Netherlands) University Medical Center at the 2011 annual meeting of the Radiological Society of North America.
15. Study author Dr Sebastiaan Hammer of the Department of Radiology at Leiden University Medical Center, presented the research in Chicago at the Radiological Society of North America's Annual Meeting, 2013. cobsnews.com, 29 November 2011. http://www.cbsnews.com/news/calorie-restriction-cures-diabetes-what-study-says.
16. Paul Dolby article, interview and quotes reported by the mailonline.co.uk, 26 December 2011.
17. S.P. Curran, X. Wu, C. Riedel and G. Ruvkun, 'A soma-to-germline transformation in long-lived Caenorhabditis elegans mutants', *Nature*, 25 June 2009, 25:459(7250):1079–84. Also see S.P. Curran, 'Conserved Mechanisms of Lifespan Regulation and Extension in *C. elegans* in Sell'; and Antonello Lorenzini, Holly M. Brown-Borg (eds), 'Life Span Extension: Single Cell Organisms to Man', *Aging Medicine*, Humana Press Inc., 2009; and Nicholas Wade, 'In Worms, Genetic Clues to Extending Longevity'. Sue McGreevey, 'Mutations extending lifespan induce expression of germline genes in somatic cells', from Massachusetts General Hospital. Brandon Keim, 'The Secret to Roundworm Longevity: Sex Cells'. Imai Shin-chiro, MD, PhD, and colleagues at the Washington University School of Medicine, 'Sirt1 extends life span and delays aging in

7. The longest-lived people in the world

1. Study by a research group at the Massachusetts General Hospital led by Sean P. Curran and Gary Ruvkun, *Nature*, 2009. Taken from two long-term study reviews based on 366,000 people aged between 18 and 59 evaluated for 22 years that was published in *JAMA*. Also see a group of calorie restrictors tested by the Washington School of Medicine and reported in the *Proceedings of the National Academy of Sciences*. **Also see** R.B. Verdery and R.L. Walford, 'Changes in plasma lipids and lipoproteins in humans during a 2-year period of dietary restriction in Biosphere T', *Archives of Internal Medicine* (*AIM*), 27 April 1998, 158(8); 900–906; and see R.L. Walford and M. Crew, 'How dietary restriction retards aging: an integrative hypothesis', *Growth, Development and Aging* (*GDA*), 1989 Winter, 53(4) 139–140.
2. Verdery, R.B. and Walford, R.L., see note 1.
3. Study by L. Fontana, 'Excessive adiposity, calorie restriction and aging in humans', *JAMA*, Vol. 293: 13, 5 April 2006.
4. Study by L.K. Heilbron, L. de Jonge, M.I. Frisard, J.P. DeLany, D. Enette, L. Meyer, J. Rood, T. Nguyen, C.K. Martin, J. Volaufova, M.M. Most, F. L. Greenway, S.R. Smith, D.A. Williamson, W.A. Deutsch and E. Ravussin, 'Effect of 6-month calorie restriction on biomarkers of aging, metabolic adaptation and oxidative stress in overweight subjects', *JAMA*, Vol. 293:13, 5 April 2006. Also study by T.E. Meyer, S.J. Kovacs, A.A. Ehsani, S. Klein, J.O. Holloszy and L. Fontana, 'Long-term caloric restriction ameliorates the decline in diastolic function in humans', *The Journal of the American College of Cardiology* (*JACC*), Vol. 47:2, pp. 398–402, 17 January 2006.
5. Study by the University of Munster, Germany, 'Caloric restriction improves memory in elderly humans', *Proceedings of the National Academy of Sciences*, February 2009.
6. 'Biological Sciences as part of the Comprehensive Assessment of Long-Term Effects of Reducing Intake of Energy conducted at the Human Nutrition Center on Aging at Tufts University', *Journal of Gerentology*, 30 April 2010. Also R.L. Walford, 'The clinical promise of dietary restriction', *Geriatrics*, April 1990, 45(4), pp. 81–83, 86–87; and study by A. Soare, R. Cangemi, D. Omedei, J.O. Holloszy and L. Fontana, 'Long-term calorie restriction, but not endurance exercise, lowers core body temperature in humans', *Aging*, Vol. 3(3), March 2011.
7. guardian.co.uk, 1 August 2010.
8. L.K. Heilbronn, L. de Jonge, M.I. Frisard *et al.*, 'Effect of 6-month calorie restriction on biomarkers of longevity, metabolic adaptation, and oxidative stress in overweight individuals: a randomized controlled trial', *JAMA*, 2006, 295(13):1539–48.
9. D.E. Larson-Meyer, B.R. Newcomer, L.K. Heilbronn *et al.*, 'Effect of 6-month calorie restriction and exercise on serum and liver lipids and markers of liver function', *Obesity* (Silver Spring), 2008,16(6):1355–62.

10. M. Franco *et al.*, 'Population-wide weight loss and regain in relation to diabetes burden and cardiovascular mortality in Cuba 1980–2010', *The British Medical Journal (BMJ)* 2013, DOI: 10.1136/bmj.f1515; and study by W.C. Willett, 'Weight changes and health in Cuba: learning from hardship', *BMJ* 2013, DOI: 10.1136/bmj.f1777, reported by MedPage Today, 9 April 2013.

11. Reported by Lee Ji-yoon, Arirang News, 10 June 2011; and englishnews@chosun.com on 22 June 2011.

12. M. Poulain, G.M. Pes, C. Grasland *et al.*, 'Identification of a geographic area characterized by extreme longevity in the Sardinia island: the AKEA study', *Experimental Gerontology*, September 2004, 39(9):1423–29. Also M. Poulain *et al.*, 'Age-Validation and Non-Random Spatial Distribution of Extreme Longevity in Sardinia: The AKEA Study', unpublished draft, November 2003.

13. M. Poulain *et al.*, 'A population where men live as long as women: Villagrande Strisaili, Sardinia', *Journal of Aging Research*, 1 December 2011, article ID 153756.

14. 'What Is Special About the Sardinian Blue Zone?', AntiAgingRemedies.org.

15. D. Reynolds, 'The Sardinian Diet May Be the Secret to Longevity', EMaxHealth.com, 21 October 2009. Also 'Blue Zone Regions – Health and Nutrition' at NutritionistWorld.com; and G.M. Pes, F. Tolu, M. Poulain *et al.*, 'Lifestyle and nutrition related to male longevity in Sardinia: an ecological study', *Nutrition, Metabolism & Cardiovascular Diseases*, 27 September 2011, doi:10.1016/j.numecd.2011.05.004.

16. Taken from the 1999 Akea project study done by the US National Institute of Aging alongside the University of Sassari on Sardinian longevity.

17. newsmaxhealth.com, 21 August 2012.

18. upi.com/health news, 6 September 2012.

19. In 2006, the Gerontological Society began identifying countries and areas where people lived the longest healthiest lives with very low disease rates and very low drug requirements. *China Daily*, 6 September 2013.

20. Statistics in this article from *The Washington Post*, 1 January 2013.

21. *ibid.*

22. Study by epidemiologist Luis Rosero-Bixby, from the University of Costa Rica in San José, and W.H. Dow, *Population Health Metrics*, 10 and 11, 2012, in *Nature*, DOI:10.1038/nature.2013.13663. Also see B.N. Uchino *et al.*, *Health Psychology 31*, 2012, pp. 789–96. Also in research by D.H. Rehkopf *et al.*, an epidemiologist at the Stanford School of Medicine in California, *Experimental Gerontology*. Also research by Michel Poulain, a demographer and longevity researcher at the Estonian Institute for Population Studies in Tallinn. Also E.S. Epel *et al.*, *Proceedings of the National Acadamy of Science of the United States of America 101*, 2004, pp. 17312–315.

23. The well-established, long-running and ongoing Adventist Health Studies, carried out by Loma Linda University, California, on 96,000 Adventists aged 30–112, from all across the USA and Canada from 1974 to the present day.

24. *ibid.*

25. B.J. Pettersen, R. Anousheh, J. Fan, K. Jaceldo-Siegl and G.E. Fraser, 'Vegetarian diets and blood pressure among white subjects: results from the Adventist Health Study-2 (AHS-2)', *Public Health Nutrition*, October 2012, 15(10).

26. Study by Greek cardiologists from the Athens University School of Medicine, conducted from June to October 2009 on over 1400 Ikarians and published in July 2011. Christina Chrysohoou, a cardiologist, told AFP that, 'While in the rest of Europe only 0.1% of the population is over 90 years old, in Ikaria the figure is tenfold, 1.1%'. Also see notes 29 and 30 and see additional notes and references on our website, www.jasonshonbennett.

27. Dr Marno Ryan from St Vincent's Hospital in Melbourne, 'The Mediterranean Diet: Improvement in Hepatic Steatosis and Insulin Sensitivity in Individuals with NAFLD'. Presented at the Liver Meeting by the American Association for the Study of Liver Diseases (AASLD) in San Francisco, 4–8 November 2011, reported by MarketWatch, 7 November 2011.

28. Study published in *The Lancet*, 2010. Researchers looked at data, including censuses, death registrations and surveys, to compile the estimated number of early deaths in 187 countries in 1970, 1990 and 2010. Reported by *BBC News*, 29 April 2010.

29. Study by researchers from the Harvard School of Public Health and the University of Athens Medical

School in Greece, covering over eight years of data from 23,000 Greek men and women participating in the European Prospective Investigation into Cancer and Nutrition (EPIC). *BMJ*, August 2013.

30. Study by researchers from the Jean Mayer USDA Human Nutrition Research Center on Aging (USDA HNRCA), the Friedman School of Nutrition Science and Policy at Tufts University, and from the CIBER Fisiopatología de la Obesidad y Nutrición, Valencia, Spain. The study was performed on 7000 PREDIMED trial patients. *Diabetes Care*, 13 August 2013. Reported by Science Codex, 13 August 2013.

31. See note 29; also further references on our website, www.jasonshonbennett.com.

32. 'The Ikaria Study', a study of 673 Ikarians by Dr Christina Chrysohoou, a cardiologist at the University of Athens' Medical School, and the Harvard School of Public Health study of 23,000 Greek adults. Reported by the *Guardian*, 31 May 2013.

33. Study by the Mayo Clinic, USA, 2013. Reported by MyHealthNewsDaily, 28 February 2013.

34. Study by Andrea Doseff, Associate Professor of Internal Medicine and Molecular Genetics at Ohio State University, and colleagues. Reported by ScienceDaily and the *Times of India*, 21 May 2013.

35. The 2013 PREDIMED Study from Spain, lead by Professor Jordi Salas-Salvadó, from the Universitat Rovira i Virgili on 7216 men and women aged 55–80.

36. Study published in *The American Journal of Clinical Nutrition*, 30 January 2013. Reported by Reuters Health, 6 February 2013.

37. Study presented to the American Heart Association in Lake Buena Vista, on 1 May 2013. Reported by WebMD News from HealthDay News, 1 May 2013.

38. As reported by the *Daily Mail*, 12 June 2013.

39. Study by Xiaoyan Huang, MD, a PhD student at the Karolinska Institute in Stockholm, Sweden. Presented to the European Renal Association-European Dialysis and Transplant Association 50th Congress in May 2013. Reported by Medscape Medical News, 21 May 2013.

40. Study from researchers at the University of Alabama at Birmingham and the University of Athens, Greece, published in *Neurology*, the medical journal of the American Academy of Neurology, May 2013. Reported by *Time Magazine*, 1 May 2013.

41. Study by Miguel A. Martinez-Gonzalez, MD, MPH, PhD, of University of Navarra, Pamplona, Spain, and colleagues, 'Mediterranean diet improves cognition: the PREDIMED-NAVARRA randomised trial'. The six-year follow-up on 552 adults, published in *The Journal of Neurology Neurosurgery and Psychiatry 2013*, DOI: 10.1136/jnnp-2013-305153. Reported by MedPage Today, 20 May 2013.

42. F. Sofi *et al.*, 'Ideal consumption for each food group composing Mediterranean Diet score for preventing total and cardiovascular mortality', presented at the European Association for Cardiovascular Prevention and Rehabilitation's EuroPRevent 2013 meeting; Abstract P106. Reported by MedPage Today, 22 April 2013.

43. M. Bes-Rastrollo, 'Costs of Mediterranean and Western dietary patterns and their relationship with prospective weight change', EuroPRevent 2013; Abstract 610. Reported by MedPage Today, 23 April 2013.

44. Study as part of the ENERGY project, published 25 April 2012 in PLoS ONE. Reported by vancouversun.com, 25 April 2012.

45. *National Geographic*, May 2013.

46. Study by T. Hofer, L. Fontana, S.D. Anton *et al.*, 'Long-term effects of caloric restriction or exercise on DNA and RNA oxidation levels in white blood cells and urine in humans', *Rejuvenation Research*, 2008, 11(4):793–99.

47. J.F. Fries, 'Japan Ministry of Health and Welfare life tables', *New England Journal of Medicine*, 1980, 303:131–35.

48. The 1976 to present day Okinawa Centenarian Study (OCS) is an ongoing population-based study of centenarians and other selected elderly in the Japanese prefecture of Okinawa that began in 1975. Also S. Mizushima *et al.*, 'The relationship of dietary factors to cardiovascular diseases among Japanese in Okinawa and Japanese immigrants, originally from Okinawa, in Brazil', *Hypertension Research*, 1992, 15:45–55.

49. *ibid.*

50. Alpa Patel of the American Cancer Society in Atlanta, and colleagues, studied 14 years of data covering over 120,000 people from the Cancer Prevention Study II Nutrition Cohort, a large,

prospective study of cancer incidence and mortality. *American Journal of Epidemiology*, 2010. Reported on 23 July 2010.

51. See note 47.
52. *ibid.*
53. *ibid.*
54. Danielle Demetriou, Tokyo and telegraph.co.uk, 4 May 2010.

8. Processed foods + overeating + overweight + obesity = short lifespan

1. Study conducted at the French National Health Institute and published in *Circulation*, February 2012, evaluated 168,159 adults who saw their primary care doctors in 63 countries across five continents in 2006. Also report by the OECD health review of 27 Asian and Pacific countries, 19 January 2011.
2. Study by Melbourne researchers Dr Cate Lombard and Professor Helena Teede of the Jean Hailes Foundation for Women's Health, *BMJ*, August 2010.
3. Study published in *Economic Inquiry*, February 2008, based on information from NHANES and the Centers for Disease Control and Prevention with contributions from the Florida State University and the Federal Reserve Bank of Boston and Diabetes Care.
4. Study of 6500 Danish men followed for 33 years by Dr Morton Schmidt and Henrik Toft Sorenson, from the Department of Clinical Epidemiology at Aarhus University Hospital in Denmark. *BMJ Open*, April 2013.
5. Study by Gerben Hulsegge from the Dutch National Institute for Public Health and the Environment, on 6000 adults aged 20–50 over a 25-year period. *The European Journal of Preventive Cardiology*, April 2013.
6. James A. Greenberg, PhD, Associate Professor, Department of Health and Nutrition Sciences at Brooklyn College of the City University of New York, 'Obesity and Early Mortality in the U.S.' The study used data from 37,632 participants in three NHANES and shows mortality is likely to occur 10–15 years earlier for the obese, *Obesity*, March 2013. Also Amy Berrington de Gonzalez *et al.*, 'Body-mass index and mortality among 1.46 million white adults', *New England Journal of Medicine*, 2012.
7. Study on peer-reviewed results, *Biodemography and Social Biology*, 2013.
8. Study data from The Physicians' Health Study, which tracked the health of 21,094 US male doctors for 20 years. *Circulation*, December 2008.
9. Michael F. Leitzmann, Corinna Koebnick, Kim N. Danforth, Louise A. Brinton, Steven C. Moore, Albert R. Hollenbeck, Arthur Schatzkin, and James V. Lacey, Jr., 'Body mass index and risk of ovarian cancer', *CANCER*, 15 February 2009. *CANCER* is a peer-reviewed journal of the American Cancer Society.
10. Australian study by Access Economics, Australian Institute of Health and Welfare, and Diabetes Australia, found that 600,000 more patients are suffering illness because of obesity than was estimated in 2006. Figure released August 2008.
11. Paul W. Franks, PhD, Robert L. Hanson, MD, MPHWilliam C. Knowler, MD, DrPH, Maurice L. Sievers, MD, Peter H. Bennett, MB, FRCP, and Helen C. Looker, MB, BS, 'Childhood Obesity, Other Cardiovascular Risk Factors, and Premature Death', *The New England Journal of Medicine*, February 2010.
12. Study published November 2007, *The American Journal of Clinical Nutrition*.
13. See note 11.
14. Study by lead researcher Andrew Renehan, of Cardiff University in Britain, as presented to the ECCO-ESMO European Cancer Congress, Berlin, September 2009, using data from the WHO and the IARC.
15. Study by the Permanente Division of Research in California, *Neurology*, November 2008.
16. Study on more than 44,000 US women tracked for over 16 years by the National Institute of Child Health and Human Development and the National Institutes of Health and Harvard Medical School. This information was presented to the American Stroke Association's International Stroke Conference 2008, from data from NHANES 1988–1994 and 1999–2004. *Circulation*, 2008.

17. Study published in *The New England Journal of Medicine*, November 2008, involved more than 350,000 people from nine countries, over ten years, and was based on research from EPIC.

18. C. Deglise *et al.*, 'Impact of obesity on diagnosis and treatment of breast cancer', *Breast Cancer Research and Treatment*, 14 July 2009. Also study by W.K. Owiredu *et al.*, 'Serum lipid profile of breast cancer patients', *Pak Journal of Biological Science*, February 2009.

19. Study on nearly 16,000 physically able, fibromyalgia-free women who were followed for 11 years, *Arthritis Care and Research*, May 2010.

20. Study by European researchers on 12,000 French men and women aged 18–69, *BMJ*, published online, June 2010.

21. Study detailed in *Human Brain Mapping*, September 2009 (online edition), funded by the National Institute on Aging, National Institute of Biomedical Imaging and Bioengineering, National Center for Research Resources, and the American Heart Association.

22. Study by Dr Diana Kerwin of Northwestern University in Chicago and colleagues, from the Women's Health Initiative data, *The Journal of the American Geriatric Society*, 14 July 2010.

23. Study by the NIH, *The Lancet*, 5 August 2010.

24. Study by Dr Frank Biro, Director of Adolescent Medicine at Cincinnati's Children's Hospital and Marcia Herman-Giddens, DrPH, PA, Adjunct Professor, Public Health, Department of Maternal and Child Health, University of North Carolina, *Pediatrics*, September 2010.

25. A 2010 New Zealand Health Ministry report on maternal and perinatal deaths released on 16 October 2010. Also see research reported in *The American Journal of Obstetrics & Gynecology*, April 2008, a study carried out at the University of Oklahoma Health Sciences Centre; and study data from the US Centres for Disease Control and Prevention's National Birth Defects Prevention research, *The American Journal of Obstetrics and Gynaecology*, October 2009.

26. Study by Harvard School of Public Health (HSPH) and Brigham Women's Hospital (BWH) from the BWH-based Nurses' Health Study, 1976 and ongoing, *BMJ*, November 2009.

27. B. Jarrett, G.J. Bloch, D. Bennett, B. Bleazard and D. Hedges, 'The influence of body mass index, age and gender on current illness: a cross-sectional study', *International Journal of Obesity*, 2010, 34:429–36, online 15 December 2009.

28. Research taken from several US mortality studies over a 30-year period and analysed by the Johns Hopkins University Medical School, 2010.

29. Study on 137 children from birth until age 28, *Journal of Pediatrics*, March 2013. Also study by the University of Jena and the German Institute of Human Nutrition, *Cell Metabolism*, August 2011.

30. Study in *JACC*, November 2012.

31. Study by lead researcher Dr Sarah Shultz, from the Institute of Health and Biomedical Innovation at the Queensland University of Technology, released at a Brisbane medical conference in November 2008.

32. Study report on US obesity rates in children by the Federal Centers for Disease Control and Prevention and The Center for Health Policy Research at the University of California at Los Angeles, released 1 August 2012.

33. From the University of Texas MD Anderson Cancer Center, reported by News.Medical.net, 22 May 2013.

34. Cari M. Kitahara, PhD, National Institutes of Health, Rockville, 'Prospective Investigation of Body Mass Index, Colorectal Adenoma, and Colorectal Cancer in the Prostate, Lung, Colorectal, and Ovarian Cancer Screening Trial' with data from the Prostate, Lung, Colorectal, and Ovarian Cancer Screening Trial. *The Journal of Clinical Oncology*, May 2013.

35. 'Overweight in Adolescence is Related to Increased Risk of Future Urothelial Cancer', a study by researchers at Tel Aviv University on 1.1 million males followed for 18 years in the National Cancer Registry. *Obesity*, 2012.

36. Study by Andrew Rundle, an Associate Professor of Epidemiology at Columbia University Mailman School of Public Health in New York City, on nearly 500 men, followed for 14 years. *Cancer Epidemiology, Biomarkers & Prevention*, 23 April 2013.

37. Study on over 400,000 Asia-Pacific people, including 10,400 New Zealanders. *The Lancet Oncology*, 30 June 2010.

38. Study by Sabrina Schlesinger at Section of Epidemiology, Institute of Experimental Medicine,

Christian-Albrechts University of Kiel in Kiel, Germany and colleagues, on 359,525 men and women enrolled in the EPIC study. *International Journal of Cancer*, September 2012.

39. Study on 1640 participants by E. Edelson, 'As obesity increases, so does stroke risk', 2010.

40. Study by K. Britton *et al.*, 'Body fat distribution, incident cardiovascular disease, cancer, and all-cause mortality'. *The Journal of the American College of Cardiology*, July 2013.

41. In 2010, a study by researchers at Johns Hopkins University of over 95,000 medical records found obesity doubles your risk of developing kidney stones.

42. A 2010 study on 13,549 middle-aged participants found that people who are obese have an increased risk of suffering from a stroke.

43. See note 41.

44. Study data from the Dutch Pediatric Surveillance Unit, published online 23 July 2012 in *The Archives of Disease in Childhood*. Also a July 2012 Centers for Disease Control and Prevention release found over 60% of obese US teens have at least one cardiovascular risk factor.

45. Study by Dr Declan O'Regan of the Medical Research Council Clinical Sciences Center at Imperial College London. *Hypertension*, June 2013.

46. Study on over 85,000 Canadians carried out by the University of Ottawa Researchers at the University of Ottawa, released April 2013.

47. *ibid.*

48. Corinna Koebnick, PhD, of Kaiser Permanente Southern California in Pasadena, and colleagues, 'Pediatric obesity and gallstone disease: results from a cross-sectional study of over 510,000 youth'. *The Journal of Pediatric Gastroenterology and Nutrition*, August 2012.

49. Alex Chang, MD *et al.*, of Johns Hopkins University, 'Lifestyle-related factors, obesity, and incident microalbuminuria: The CARDIA study'. *The American Journal of Kidney Disease*, April 2013.

50. F.X. Castellanos *et al.*, 'Obesity in men with childhood ADHD: a 33-year controlled, prospective follow-up study', at the Child Study Center at NYU Langone Medical Center. *Pediatrics* (online edition), 20 May 2013.

51. Study by Paresh Dandona, MD, PhD, SUNY, Muniza Mogri, MD; Husam Ghanim, PhD and Teresa Quattrin, MD. *Clinical Endocrinology* (online edition), October, 2012.

52. E.S. Epel, J. Lin, F.H. Wilhelm *et al.*, 'Cell aging in relation to stress arousal and cardiovascular disease risk factors'. *Psychoneuroendocrinology*, 2006, 31(3):277. Also see The Bogalusa Heart Study by J.P. Gardner, S. Li, S.R. Srinivasan *et al.*, 'Rise in insulin resistance is associated with escalated telomere attrition'. *Circulation*, 2005, 111:2171–77.

53. Quotes by Katie Bayne, Coca-Cola's president of sparkling beverages in North America, were taken directly from the interview she gave with the *Detroit Free Press* and *USA Today*, published 8 June 2012.

54. Miller, Jake, 'Weight and mortality: Researchers challenge results of obesity analysis'. *Overweight and Obesity (Medical Xpress)*, 25 February 2013. Also see P. De Wal *et al.*, 'Reviews on sugar-sweetened beverage and body weight: Determinants of their quality and conclusions', presented at the European Congress on Obesity, Liverpool, May 2013.

55. Study conducted by researchers from Kaleida Health in Buffalo, New York. *Journal of Clinical Endocrinology & Metabolism*, September 2012.

56. Study conducted by researchers at the VU University Amsterdam (the Netherlands), *The New England Journal of Medicine*, 2013. The study used data from three previous studies: the Nurses' Health Study, the Health Professionals Follow-up Study and the Women's Genome Health Study.

57. Study by researchers at the University of Sydney covering over 2000 12-year-olds. Reported by The Australian Broadcasting Corporation and WebMD Health News on 4 April 2012.

58. Study conducted on 224 overweight adolescents at Children's Hospital Boston, results released March 2013.

59. Z. Shi *et al.*, 'Association between soft drink consumption and asthma and chronic obstructive pulmonary disease among adults in Australia'. *Respirology*, 7 February 2012.

60. Study published online by *The New England Journal of Medicine*, October 2012. The study used results of over 33,000 American men and women.

61. See note 56.

62. Study by Eric J. Jacobs, PhD, Christina C. Newton, MSPH, Yiting Wang, PhD, Alpa V. Patel, PhD, Marjorie L. McCullough, ScD, Peter T. Campbell, PhD, Michael J. Thun, MD and Susan M. Gapstur,

PhD. 'Waist Circumference and All-Cause Mortality in a Large US Cohort'. *The Archives of Internal Medicine*, August 2010, 170(15):1293–1301.

63. Numbers taken from the highly regarded 'Comprehensive Assessment of the Long Term Effects of Reducing Intake of Energy (CALERIE)' study.

9. A plant-based wholefood diet + Regular Intelligent Fasting® = a long healthy life

1. Study by Tasnime Akbaraly, PhD, *et al.*, of INSERM in Montpellier, France, 'Does overall diet in midlife predict future aging phenotypes? A cohort study'. American Heart Association, *The American Journal of Medicine*, May 2013, 126:411–19.
2. Study results by Haitham Ahmed and researchers at the Ciccarone Center for the Prevention of Heart Disease, from the multi-center Multi-Ethnic Study of Atherosclerosis (MESA). *The American Journal of Epidemiology*, 3 June 2013.
3. Study on more than 200,000 adults in the US aged 50 to 71 over a period of 11 years, conducted by the National Heart, Lung, and Blood Institute at the National Institutes of Health. Released to the public on 18 November 2011.
4. From studies published in *JAMA*, Vol. 295, pp. 1539–48), US National Institute on Aging in Baltimore. Also published works and comments from *Nature Medicine*, Auckland University's Department of Molecular Medicine and Pathology; and the Brain and Behaviour Research Group at Britain's Open University.
5. Study in *The Journal of Clinical Endocrinology Metabolism*, April 2010.
6. A 2011 study from the Medical College of Georgia, Augusta.
7. Study conducted by Harvard Medical School on some 40,000 American women, results released March 2013.
8. Study by Sun Ha Jee, carried out by Johns Hopkins Bloomberg School of Public Health and Yonsei University in Seoul, Korea. The study followed almost 1.3 million Korean men and women, aged between 30 and 95 years, from 2001 to 2011. Also see a study on more than 50,000 men at Harvard University, released January 2013.
9. Study on almost 78,000 Swedish men and women carried out by Karolinska Institute in Stockholm, Sweden and Central Hospital in Västerås, Sweden. Results released April 2013.
10. The Iowa Women's Health Study on 23,000 post-menopausal women, 2011. Also an Italian endometrial cancer study and a Washington University School of Medicine in Missouri Study as released 2010. 11. Study published by the Rudd Center for Food Policy and Obesity at Yale University, with 4000 people responding to an online survey about obesity. Results released February 2012.
12. M. Winick *et al.*, *Childhood Obesity*, Wiley, New York, 1975. Also, body weight is influenced by genes but your size is more influenced by diet and lifestyle, as shown on 'The Great British Body: DNA testing', reported by the *New Zealand Herald*, 16 November 2010.
13. Study by T. Gordon and W.B. Kannel. *Geriatrics*, 1973, 28:80.
14. Research from the five-year study of 300 children by Peninsula Medical School in the UK was presented to the European Congress on Obesity. *Occupational and Environmental Medicine*, July 2012.
15. A study by British scientists from Peninsula Medical School at the universities of Exeter and Plymouth. Reported by AAP, 14 July 2009.
16. Study by researchers from the University of Western Australia, and Perth's Telethon Institute for Child Health Research. *Diabetes Care*, January 2009.
17. Study by Esther Zimmermann, PhD, of the Institute of Preventive Medicine in Copenhagen University.

10. Weight-loss drugs and weight-loss surgery

1. 'Weight Loss/Obesity Management Market Global Forecasts to 2017' Report, May 2013.
2. Study by Professor Sabine Rohrmann, Professor of Epidemiology, University of Zurich, and a multinational group of scientists, on 448,568 people in ten European countries as published in

BioMed Central (*BMC*) *Medicine*, on 6 March 2013; Also see 'Vascular effects of a low-carbohydrate high-protein diet', released by Harvard Medical School, 17 July 2009; Also see W.C. Miller *et al.*, *Growth*, 1984:48:415; Also J. Kaluza *et al.*, 'Red meat consumption and risk of stroke: a meta-analysis of prospective studies', a 329,495 participant study as published in *Stroke: Journal of the American Heart* Association, in August 2012. Also A. Pan *et al.*, 'Red Meat Consumption and Risk of Type 2 Diabetes: 3 Cohorts of U.S. Adults and an Updated Meta-Analysis'; Also 'Meats, processed meats, obesity, weight gain and occurrence of diabetes among adults: findings from Adventist Health Studies', *Annals of Nutrition and Metabolism*, 2008:52(2):96–104 and 2010:56(3):232.

3. Study conducted by Brazilian and Canadian researchers and published in the *BMJ*, 2010.

4. Study by Dr M. Maggard-Gibbons M *et al.*, 'Bariatric surgery for weight loss and glycemic control in non-morbidly obese adults with diabetes: a systematic review', *JAMA*, 5 June 2013, 309:2250–61. Also see a study by a team at the University of Colorado, *Obesity*, 2011.

5. *ibid*; also see additional notes and references on our website, www.jasonshonbennett.com.

6. Research from the University of California, San Diego, reported by the *Daily Mail*, 6 July 2010. Also see additional notes and references on our website, www.jasonshonbennett.com.

7. A.P. Liou *et al.*, 'Conserved shifts in the gut microbiota due to gastric bypass reduce host weight and adiposity', *Science Translational Medicine*, 2013:5:178ra41, 27 March 2013.

8. Study conducted at the Washington University School of Medicine in Missouri investigating the digestive tract of fat and thin people, May 2011.

9. M. Zupancic *et al.*, 'Analysis of the gut microbiota in the Old Order Amish and its relation to the metabolic syndrome'. PLoS One, 2012, DOI:10.1371/journal.pone.0043052, 15 August 2012.

10. Reported by the editors of *Environmental Nutrition Newsletter*, Premium Health News Service, 10 October 2012.

11. J. Zimmer, B. Lange *et al.*, 'A vegan or vegetarian diet substantially alters the human colonic faecal microbiota'. *European Journal of Clinical Nutrition 2012*, vol. 66, pp. 53–60, DOI:10.1038/ejcn.2011.141.

12. *ibid*.

13. Study co-authored by biochemist and PhD student Jan-Hendrik Hehemann at the Station Biologique de Roscoff in France. *Nature*, April 2010.

14. Report published in *BMC Nutrition*, May 2012.

15. NZ Government statistics. Also see National Cancer Registry (2008); and Colorectal Cancer Registrations by Year and DHB figures. By 2016 the number of new cases of bowel cancer diagnosed each year is projected to increase by 15% for men and 19% for women.

16. Study by Dr Evropi Theodoratou, of the University of Edinburgh's School of Molecular, Genetic and Population Health Sciences. *The European Journal of Cancer Prevention*, 14 July 2013.

17. 'Prospective Investigation of Body Mass Index, Colorectal Adenoma, and Colorectal Cancer in the Prostate, Lung, Colorectal, and Ovarian Cancer Screening Trial', with data from the Prostate, Lung, Colorectal, and Ovarian Cancer Screening Trial, by Cari M. Kitahara, PhD, of the *NIH* in Rockville. *The Journal of Clinical Oncology*, May 2013.

18. Study released jointly by the World Cancer Research Fund, the American Institute for Cancer Research and the European Prospective Investigation of Cancer, covering more than 500,000 participants, July 2012.

19. A. Bellavia, S.C. Larsson, M. Bottai, A. Wolk and N. Orsini, 'Fruit and vegetable consumption and all-cause mortality: a dose-response analysis'. A Swedish study published in *The American Journal of Clinical Nutrition* (online), 26 June 2013.

20. *ibid*.

21. Study by a team of scientists from the US, Tanzania and the UK. PLoS ONE, 26 July 2012.

22. The 2012 IHME Report, 12 July 2013. Also see a study released 10 April 2012 by Brazil's Health Ministry on up-to-date data from 2011 Health Ministry surveys of 54,144 people in the capitals of Brazil's 27 states.

23. Report by the *Canadian Medical Association Journal*, March 2009.

24. Studies by the Physical Activity and Weight Management Research Centre at the University of Pittsburgh, and by Timothy Church, Director of the Laboratory of Preventive Medicine at the Pennington Biomedical Research Centre in Louisiana, February 2012.

25. A study by the American Academy of Sleep Medicine in *Sleep* (online), 1 May 2012. Reported by *Today* on 1 May 2012.

11. Eat less, eat better, move more, have a rhythm, live long

1. A 2009 National Institute on Aging Pew Research Center poll of 2969 American adults.
2. Study published in the *Proceedings of the National Academy of Sciences* with research from the Preventive Medicine Research Institute in Sausalito, California, 17 June 2008.
3. J.P. Gardner, S. Li, S.R. Srinivasan *et al.*, 'Rise in insulin resistance is associated with escalated telomere attrition'. The Bogalusa Heart Study, *Circulation*, 2005, 111:2171–77.
4. Study by Andrew Dillin of the Salk Institute for Biological Studies in La Jolla, *Nature*, June 2009. Also see news from *The Scientist*, 2003, 4(1):20030124-02 DOI:10.1186/20030124-02 Science, 299:572–574, 24 January 2003; and 2001, 2(1):20010831-02.
5. Kim Severson, *Mind over Platter*. Reported in the *New York Times* and reprinted in the *Sydney Morning Herald*, 13 November 2008.
6. Ivan Araujo, Albino Oliviera-Maia, Tatyana Sotnikova, Raul Gainetdinov, Marc Caron, Miguel Nicolelis, Sidney Simon, 'Food reward in the absence of taste receptor signaling'. *Neuron*, DOI:10.1016/j.neuron.2008.01.032.
7. *New Scientist*, 2 September 2010.
8. 'Brain Pathway Responsible For Obesity Found: Too Many Calories Send Brain Off Kilter'. *Cell*, 2 October 2008. Also see 'How Fatty Foods Curb Hunger', University of California, *ScienceDaily*, 7 October 2008.
9. 'The Secrets of Long Life,' based on worldwide research by Dan Buettner. *National Geographic Magazine*, May 2012.
10. University of Illinois study. *Obesity*, 2011.
11. Study by Duk-Hee Lee and an international team of colleagues at the Kyungpook National University in Daegu in South Korea, on 1099 Americans. *International Journal of Obesity*, September 2010.

13. Why fast?

1. Study by Markus Stoffel, Professor at the Institute of Molecular Systems Biology at ETH Zurich. *Nature*, December 2009.
2. Study by Greek cardiologists from the Athens University School of Medicine, conducted June–October 2009 on over 1400 of Ikaria's 8000 residents, divided into elderly and middle-aged groups and assessing lifestyle, diet, clinical and other factors. Published in July 2011.

15. Fasting, the liver, and your skin

1. Study and quotes from Dr Chhabra and Dr John Helzberg, presentation at the 2013 American Gastroenterological Association annual meeting. Reported by Health24.com, 25 June 2013.
2. Dr Paul Trembling and Professor William Rosenberg, UCL Institute of Liver and Digestive Health, 'Influence of BMI and alcohol on liver-related morbidity and mortality in a cohort of 108,000 women from the general population from UKCTOCS; Abstract 115'. Presented at the 2013 International Liver Congress, The Netherlands, 25 April 2013..
3. Study by J.S. Allard, L.K. Heilbronn, C. Smith *et al.*, the Kronos Longevity Research Institute. PLoS ONE, 2008, 3(9):e3211.
4. Research by Amy Walker, PhD, the MGH Cancer Center, and investigators at Massachusetts General Hospital. *Genes & Development*, 2010.

16. Fasting and weight loss

1. Study by H. Norrelund *et al.*, 'The protein-retaining effects of growth hormone during fasting involve inhibition of muscle-protein breakdown'. *Diabetes*, January 2001, Vol. 50:1, pp. 96–104. Also H. Norrelund, 'The metabolic role of growth hormone in humans with particular reference to fasting.' *Growth Hormone & IGF Research*, 15(2):95–122, April 2005; and a study conducted by Benjamin

D. Horne, PhD, MPH, Director of Cardiovascular and Genetic Epidemiology at the Intermountain Medical Center Heart Institute, Salt Lake City, and colleagues in the Intermountain Medical Center Heart Institute research team. Presented at the annual scientific sessions of the American College of Cardiology, New Orleans, 2011.

2. Study by Krista A. Varady, Surabhi Bhutani, Emily C. Church and Monica C. Klempel, supported by the Department of Kinesiology and Nutrition, University of Illinois at Chicago, Chicago, Illinois, and by departmental funding from the University of Illinois at Chicago. Registered at clinicaltrials.gov as UIC-004-2009, 12 July 2009.

3. Study by Matthew D. Bruss, Cyrus F. Khambatta, Ishita Aggarwal and Marc K. Hellerstein, Department of Nutritional Sciences and Toxicology, University of California at Berkeley, Berkeley, and Maxwell A. Ruby from Children's Hospital Oakland Research Institute, Oakland, California. Published 2 November 2009.

4. Human Nutrition Unit at the University of Aberdeen Rowett Institute of Nutrition and Health scientists, 'Metabolomics of prolonged fasting in humans reveals new catabolic markers'. *Metabolomics*, DOI: 10.1007/s11306-010-0255-2.

5. J. Gjedsted *et al.*, 'Effects of a 3-day fast on regional lipid and glucose metabolism in human skeletal muscle and adipose tissue'. *Acta Physiologica*, Vol. 191:3 pp. 205–16.

6. Study by M.N. Harvie, M. Pegington, M.P. Mattson, J. Frystyk, B. Dillon, G. Evans, J. Cuzick, S.A. Jebb, B. Martin, R.G. Cutler, T.G. Son, S. Maudsley, O.D. Carlson, J.M. Egan, A. Flyvbjerg and A. Howell from the Genesis Prevention Centre, University Hospital of South Manchester, NHS Foundation Trust, Manchester, UK. *International Journal of Obesity* (advance online version), 5 October 2010. Also see a randomised, controlled trial with 81 adults with metabolic syndrome, presented at the Experimental Biology Meeting, April 2009.

7. The study was a randomised, controlled trial of 81 adults with metabolic syndrome overseen by Baylor College of Medicine. Results showed than a daily intake of an 8-ounce glass of juice as part of a calorie-controlled DASH diet led to a 4-pound reduction in weight over 12 weeks, while those that followed the same diet but drank no juice lost 1 pound. Researchers found that participants in the group that took vegetable juice while watching their calorie intake were more likely to meet the daily five-a-day recommendation for fruit and vegetable intake. 'What this study shows is that by taking simple, proactive steps such as drinking low sodium vegetable juice while watching calorie intake, people can begin to control their weight, which helps reduce the risk of long-term health implications,' said study author John Foreyt, PhD. The results of the study were presented at the Experimental Biology Meeting, April 2009.

8. Study by C. O'Neil *et al.*, 'A Review of the Relationship Between 100% Fruit Juice Consumption and Weight in Children and Adolescents'. *American Journal of Lifestyle Medicine*, 2008, vol. 2, no. 4, pp. 315–54. Also see T. Nicklas, C. O'Neil and R. Kleinman, 'Association Between 100% Juice Consumption and Nutrient Intake and Weight of Children Aged 2 to 11 Years'. *Archives of Pediatric and Adolescent Medicine*, 2008, 162(6), pp.557–65. T.A. Nicklas, C.E. O'Neil, and R. Kleinman, 'The Relationship Among 100% Juice Consumption, Nutrient Intake, and Weight of Adolescents 12 to 18 Years'. Presented at annual scientific meeting of The North American Association for the Study of Obesity, New Orleans, Louisiana, October 2007. Also Abstract No. 538-P, containing data collected from the National Health and Nutrition Examination survey between 1999 and 2004.

9. Study by U. Leuven, Tervuursevest, K. Van Proeyen, K. Szlufcik, H. Nielens, M. Ramaekers, and P. Hespel. The Research Centre for Exercise and Health, FaBeR-K, the *Journal of Applied Physiology*, January 2011, 110(1):236–45.

10. D.T. Kirkendall, J.B. Leiper, Z. Bartagi, J. Dvorak and Y. Zerguini, 'The influence of Ramadan fasting on physical performance measures in young Muslim footballers' at the FIFA Medical Assessment and Research Centre, Schulthess Clinic, Zurich, Switzerland. The *Journal of Sports Science*, 26 December 2008, Suppl.3:S15–27.

11. K. De Bock, W. Derave, B.O. Eijnde, M.K. Hesselink, E. Koninckx, A.J. Rose, P. Schrauwen, A. Bonenand E.A. Richter, 'Effect of training in the fasted state on metabolic responses during exercise with carbohydrate intake'. The *Journal of Applied Physiology*, April 2008. Also see the *Journal of Applied Physiology*, June 2009, 106(6):1757–58.

17. The science of fasting

1. A Norwegian study by Jens Kjeldsen-Kragh *et al*, 2006.
2. Study published in *Science*, May/June 2008 from research at the Harvard Medical School. Reuters.
3. Study published in *Free Radical Biology & Medicine*, 2007.
4. Study lead by Dr James Johnson, at Louisiana State University, 2010. Reported on 13 February 2010.
5. Dr Max Gerson. *A Cancer Therapy – Fifty Case Histories*. Whittier Beeks, NYC. Distributed by Cancer Book House, 2043 N. Berendo Street, Los Angeles, California.
6. Study published in the *Proceedings of the National Academy of Sciences*, using data from a study done by the University of Southern California, April 2008. Also see 'Fasting Cycles Retard Growth of Tumors and Sensitize a Range of Cancer Cell'. *Science Translational Medicine Rapid Publication*, 8 February 2012, DOI: 10.1126/scitranslmed.3003293.
7. *ibid.*
8. Study published in *Science Translational Medicine*, 8 February 2012, reported 10 February 2012. Also see J.S. Allard, L.K. Helibronn, C. Smith *et al.*, 'In vitro cellular adaptations of indicators of longevity in response to treatment with serum collected from humans on calorie restricted diets.'
9. Fernando M. Safdie, Tanya Dorff, David Quinn, Luigi Fontana, Min Wei, Changhan Lee, Pinchas Cohen, and Valter D. Longo, 'Fasting and cancer treatment in humans: A case series report'. *Aging*, Vol. 1, No. 12, 31 December 2009. Also see Changhan Lee, Fernando M. Safdie, Lizzia Raffaghello, Min Wei, Federica Madia, Edoardo Parrella, David Hwang, Pinchas Cohen, Giovanna Bianchi, and Valter D. Longo, 'Reduced Levels of IGF-I Mediate Differential Protection of Normal and Cancer Cells in Response to Fasting and Improve Chemotherapeutic Index'. *Cancer Research*, Vol. 70, No. 4, 15 February 2010.
10. Study published in *Cancer Research*, January 2010. Also see 'Fasting Cycles Retard Growth of Tumors and Sensitize a Range of Cancer Cell'. *Science Translational Medicine Rapid Publication*, DOI: 10.1126/scitranslmed.3003293, 8 February 2012.
11. N. Halberg *et al.*, 'Effect of intermittent fasting and refeeding on insulin action in healthy men'. *Journal of Applied Physiology*, 99:2128–36, 2005. Also see study in *Nature*, 8 April 2012. Also L. Heilbronn, S.R. Smith and E. Ravussin, 'Failure of fat cell proliferation, mitochondrial function and fat oxidation results in ectopic fat storage, insulin resistance and type II diabetes mellitus'. *International Journal of Obesity and Metabolic Disorders*, 2004, 28(suppl):S12–21. Also new research presented on 3–5 April 2011 at the Annual Sientific Sessions of the American College of Cardiology in New Orleans, by Benjamin D. Horne, PhD, MPH, Director of Cardiovascular and Genetic Epidemiology at the Intermountain Medical Center Heart Institute in Salt Lake City. Also L.K. Heilbronn, A.E. Civitarese, I. Bogacka, S.R. Smith, M. Hulver and E. Ravussin, 'Glucose tolerance and skeletal muscle gene expression in response to alternate day fasting'. *Obesity Research*, 2005, 13:574–81. Also a study that found a striking preventative association between fasting and heart disease among 448 patients, *American Journal of Cardiology*, 2008. Also L.K. Heilbronn, S.R. Smith, C.K. Martin, S.D. Anton and E. Ravussin, 'Alternate-day fasting in non-obese subjects: effects on body weight, body composition, and energy metabolism'. *American Journal of Clinical Nutrition*, 2005, 81:69–73. Also 'Routine periodic fasting found to be good for heart health'. Presented by Intermountain Medical Center scientists at the American College of Cardiology in New Orleans, April 2011.
12. *ibid.*
13. *ibid.*
14. *ibid.*
15. Study by American researchers looking at nationwide health data from 1999–2004. The study found juice drinkers were generally leaner and they had better insulin sensitivity, which reduced the risk of stroke, heart disease and diabetes. Reported by Fairfax, April 2009.
16. Study by the University of California at Davis, presented at the annual conference of the American Dietetic Association, November 2008, Chicago. Also see a Vanderbilt University research team study published in the *American Journal of Medicine*. Also study in *Biomedical Environmental Science*, February 2008. Also study by Latvian scientists, *Planta Medica*, 2008.
17. D. Hay, *Cardiovascular Disease in New Zealand. 2004. A Summary of Recent Statistical Information*. 2004. Also see *Key Results of the 2006/07 New Zealand Health Survey*. The National Heart Foundation of New Zealand, Ministry of Health, 2008.

18. The 12-year study by doctors affiliated with TrueNorth Health Education Center and completed in conjunction with Cornell University. *Journal of Manipulative and Physiological Therapeutics*, vol. 24, no. 5, June 2001. Also see study published in the *Journal of Alternative and Complementary Medicine*, October 2002. Also see study by Dr Benjamin D. Horne, Intermountain Medical Center in Salt Lake City. Presented at the American Heart Association's Scientific Sessions, Florida, November 2007.

19. *ibid.*

20. Amrita Ahluwalia, PhD *et al.*, Queen Mary University of London, 'Enhanced vasodilator activity of nitrite in hypertension: critical role for erythrocytic xanthine oxidoreductasse and translational potential'. Funded by the British Heart Foundation. *Hypertension: Journal of the American Heart Association*, 2013. Reported by MedPage Today, 15 April 2013.

21. Study presented by researchers from Intermountain Medical Center and the University of Utah at a conference of the American Heart Association, July 2008.

22. Benjamin D. Horne, PhD, MPH, Jeffrey L. Anderson, MD, John F. Carlquist, PhD, J. Brent Muhlestein, MD, Donald L. Lappé, MD, Heidi T. May, PhD, MSPH, Boudi Kfoury, MD, Oxana Galenko, PhD, Amy R. Butler, Dylan P. Nelson, Kimberly D. Brunisholz, Tami L. Bair, and Samin Panahi, 'Routine periodic fasting found to be good for heart health'. Reported by media 3–5 April 2011; presented at the annual 2011 Scientific Sessions of the American College of Cardiology, reported in DiabetesHealth.com, 6 May 2011.

23. Trial study carried out by Dr Krista Varady, the University of California and the University of Illinois, Chicago, on the long-term effects of fasting. Also see a 2013 study by Chief Interventional Cardiologist Dr Omar Hallak at the American Hospital Dubai. Reported by pakistantoday.com, 8 July 2013.

24. Kelly Décorde, P.-L. Teissèdre, C. Auger, J.-P. Cristol, J.-M. Rouanet, the University of Montpellier 1 and 2, and the Victor Ségalen University in Bordeaux 2,'Phenolics from purple grape, apple, purple grape juice and apple juice prevent early atherosclerosis induced by an atherogenic diet in hamsters'. *Molecular Nutrition & Food Research*, 2008, DOI:10.1002/mnfr.200700141, vol. 52, pp. 400–407.

25. Andrew J. Webb, N. Patel, S. Loukogeorgakis, M. Okorie, Z. Aboud, S. Misra, R. Rashid, P. Miall, J. Deanfield, N. Benjamin, R. MacAllister, A.J. Hobbs, and A. Ahluwalia, 'Acute blood pressure lowering, vasoprotective and anti-platelet properties of dietary nitrate via bioconversion to nitrite'. *Hypertension*, March 2008, 51(3), pp. 784–90. Also see the editorial in the *Journal of the American Heart Association: Hypertension*, 4 February 2008. Also D.A. Wink and N. Paolocci, 'Mother Was Right: Eat Your Vegetables and Do Not Spit! When Oral Nitrate Helps With High Blood Pressure'. *Journal of the American Heart Association: Hypertension*, February 2008.

26. A.A. Haghdoost and M. Poorranjbar, Physiology Research Center, Kerman University of Medical Sciences, Jomhoori Islamic Boulevard, Kerman 7618747653, Iran, *Singapore Medical Journal*, 50(9):897–901, September 2009.

27. S. Bhutani, M.C. Klempel, R.A. Berger, K.A. Varady KA, Department of Kinesiology and Nutrition, University of Illinois at Chicago, Chicago, Illinois, USA. *Obesity* (Silver Spring), 18(11):2152–920, 10 November, Epub, 18 March 2010.

28. Study published in *Nutrition Journal*, December 2012. Also see a study published in the *British Journal of Nutrition*, March 2012. The study showed that beetroot juice was able to reduce blood pressure in a group of 18 men in as little as three hours. Reported by Learning from New and AFP Relax News, 18 December 2012. Also see Amrita Ahluwalia, PhD *et al.*, Queen Mary University of London, 'Enhanced vasodilator activity of nitrite in hypertension: critical role for erythrocytic xanthine oxidoreductasse and translational potential'. Funded by the British Heart Foundation. *Hypertension: Journal of the American Heart Association*, 2013. Reported by MedPage Today, 15 April 2013.

29. 'Effect of potentially modifiable risk factors associated with myocardial infarction in 52 countries (the INTERHEART study): case-control study'. *The Lancet*, 2004, 364:937–952. Also A. Rosengren, S. Hawken, S. Ounpuu *et al.*, for the INTERHEART investigators, 'Association of psychosocial risk factors with risk of acute myocardial infarction in 11 119 cases and 13 648 controls from 52 countries (the INTERHEART study): case-control study'. *The Lancet*, 2004, 364:953–962. Also see M. Ezzati, 'How can cross-country research on health risks strengthen interventions? Lessons from INTERHEART'. *The Lancet*, 2004, 364:912–914. Also studies by S. Yusuf, S. Hawken, S. Ounpuu, on

behalf of the INTERHEART Study Investigators, *INTERHEART: A Global Case-Control Study of Risk Factors for Acute Myocardial Infarction.* This major Canadian-led global study was a standardised case-control study at 262 participating centres in 52 countries throughout Africa, Asia, Australia, Europe, the Middle East, and North and South America.

30. See note 27.
31. Study published by the American Association for the Advancement of Science (AAAS), 3 April 2011.
32. *New Scientist*, November 2012.
33. The study, published in *Nutrition Research*, by the University College Cork.
34. Study by researchers at Fred Hutchinson Cancer Research Center. The research was supported by a NIH Ruth L. Kirschstein National Research Service Award, the American Diabetes Association and the National Institute of Diabetes and Digestive and Kidney Diseases. *Science*, 2009; reported in ScienceDaily, 28 August 2009.
35. www.news-medical, 21 July 2008.

18. Preparation for fasting

1. Study carried out at the School of Psychology, Hertfordshire University. *Appetite*, May 2008.
2. Food cravings and stress study carried out by scientists at the University of California.
3. Ivan Araujo, Albino Oliviera-Maia, Tatyana Sotnikova, Raul Gainetdinov, Marc Caron, Miguel Nicolelis, Sidney Simon with research from Duke University Medical Center in Durham, North Carolina, 'Food reward in the absence of taste receptor signalling'. *Neuron*, DOI: 10.1016/j.neuron.2008.01.032.

Appendix: Centenarians tell their secrets

1. *Washington Post*, 3 January 2013.
2. Reported from London and by newstrackindia.com, 9 March 2013, *The Times of India*, ANI.
3. As reported on 7 July 2012.
4. Alison Hunt and Audrey Duthie celebrated their hundredth birthday on 8 August 2010. *New Zealand Herald*, 5 August 2010.
5. Reported by Scott Herhold in MercuryNews.com, 15 March 2010.
6. Reported by Sue Scheible in *The Patriot Ledger*, 22 March 2010.
7. Reported by Jerry Robinson in *The Highline Times*, 22 March 2010.
8. Reported by Reuters, 23 May 2013.
9. *New Hanover County News*, August 2010.
10. Reported by *The New York Times, Herald-Tribune*, 11 July 2012.

Please send me your adventures, fasting experiences, feedback and thoughts at info@jasonshonbennett.com.

If you enjoyed this book and you are

a) genuinely interested in getting well and staying well,

b) looking for support and expertise while you get well, and

c) discovering that a real education about health is appealing to you,

you may be interested in finding out more about my educational work.

Visit www.jasonshonbennett.com for information about our seminars, weekend workshops, fasting retreats, and thelifeplan®.

We are also accessible through my blog, Facebook and YouTube. You can also listen to one of my CDs or watch a DVD.

Above all, look after yourself and your family and make sure you eat well, get well and stay well.

Thank you so much for your time and for placing your faith in me.

Jason